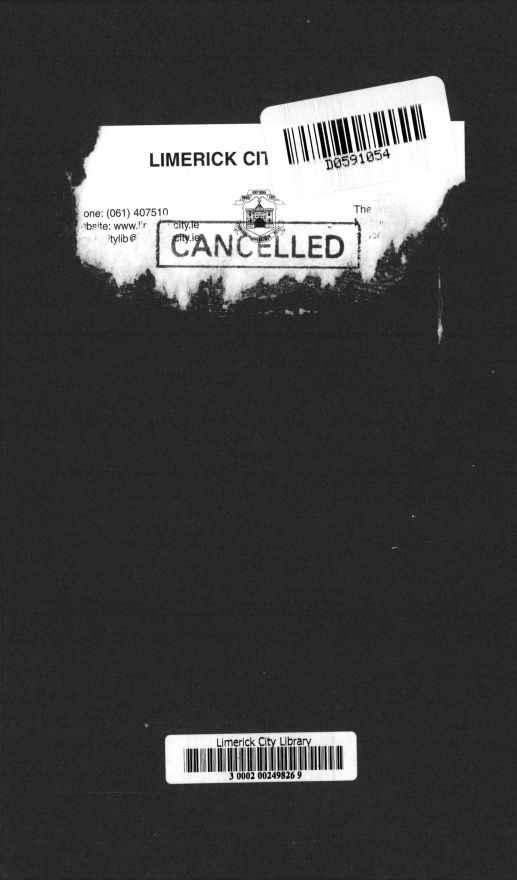

Flesh and Blood

Books are frequently dedicated to the memory of a loved one.
I dedicate mine to the living:

the dreams and inspiration of my late husband,
Stephen Brian Blood 1965 – 1995

and our wonderful children,
Liam Stephen Blood born 1998
and
Joel Michael Blood born 2002

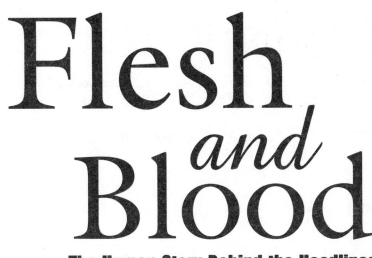

Flesh and Blood

The Human Story Behind the Headlines

DIANE BLOOD

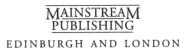

CANCELLED

MAINSTREAM
PUBLISHING
EDINBURGH AND LONDON

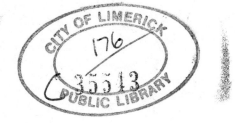

First published in Great Britain in 2004 by
MAINSTREAM PUBLISHING COMPANY (EDINBURGH) LTD
7 Albany Street
Edinburgh EH1 3UG

ISBN 1 84018 911 8

Lyrics from 'Two Worlds' on pp. 259–61 reproduced by kind permission
of Heaven and Earth Music. Lyrics written by Craig Pruess.
www.heaven-on-earth-music.co.uk

A catalogue record for this book is available from the British Library

Typeset in Baskerville Book
Printed and bound in Great Britain by
Mackays of Chatham plc

CONTENTS

FOREWORD

This is a story of a very brave woman. But it is a story that should really never have needed to be told, about a bitter battle that should never have taken place. It is a story about the inflexibility of some powerful people who felt they were serving some public purpose, and the remarkable persistence of a solitary widow who simply sought justice after the tragic premature death of her husband. This grieving woman, poignantly and against the odds, stood against the mighty British Establishment and persisted in a fight to have her husband's child – a child that both she and her husband, Stephen, had long planned.

It all started with meningitis. After a sudden, brutally short illness, Stephen Blood died. During his last few days in Intensive Care, sperm was taken from him for frozen preservation. It had always been his express wish that Diane should have his child in the event of his death, and, as a religious individual, Diane gave approval for his sperm to be stored. She wanted to fulfil what she was certain was Stephen's dying resolve. And the British regulatory body, the Human Fertilisation and Embryology Authority (HFEA), established by the Government to supervise embryo research and various aspects of fertility treatment, gave their authorisation so that sperm storage could take place.

But months later, when it came to the crunch, the HFEA suddenly seemed to change course. They refused permission for Diane Blood to use the stored sperm taken from her dead husband. They invoked the precise wording of the law, arguing that, because Stephen was too ill to have actually physically signed consent for sperm storage and insemination, Diane could not have his child. Ironically, she could try for a baby using donated sperm from any individual anonymously chosen from a sperm bank. But even with the full support of her dead husband's family, Diane could not carry out what she believed to be Stephen's dearest wish.

What followed is, in my view, a blot on the history of the Government's regulatory authority. When Diane's expensive and lengthy legal action to get permission to use the semen failed, the HFEA seemed almost vindictive. They justified their actions in the broadcast media and even pursued Diane for the HFEA's legal costs. With the frenzy in the newspapers that inevitably followed, some members of the HFEA clearly took the view that Diane was simply doing all this for the publicity. In fact, all she wanted was a just settlement with personal privacy. Some of the regulators stated privately that they were upholding an important principle against somebody who, to some of them, appeared somewhat deranged. But what public good could possibly be served by refusing Diane Blood treatment remained obscure.

Diane Blood, her family and her legal advisers remained steadfast. After a lengthy and costly process in the Court of Appeal, a legal ruling gave Diane a tiny loophole – whilst saving the face of the HFEA. Diane Blood could legally export her husband's frozen semen samples to a country in the European Union, providing the HFEA approved. After a little further negotiation, the HFEA backed down, and it was agreed that the best place for Diane's treatment would be Brussels in Belgium. There the doctors had an excellent track record using IVF with stored sperm samples.

The Belgian treatment (which could so easily have been carried out without charge in the UK) was successful. Liam Blood, a delightful little boy, is now five years old. And his younger brother Joel was born just two years ago in July 2002, after Diane went through a further course of treatment. Nobody now can doubt the wonder of the existence of these children, nor the delight they give to Stephen Blood's whole family. Very few people now feel that Diane's resolve to pursue treatment was other than totally justified. It is clear to all that it has ended entirely happily.

Diane's story is most moving. But it also raises some very important social questions, particularly about the way modern society is often regulated. Our society is increasingly tightly controlled, and sometimes huge power is given to those who are appointed to enforce the regulations. Why should 'consent for treatment' necessarily always be in writing, as the HFEA in obeying the letter of the law was required to rule? To what extent should 'right-thinking' people decide what Diane and her husband had personally agreed? And how can the 'Establishment' determine what is in the best interests of an unborn child? Should private individuals be able to decide what is right for them when their decision cannot threaten the moral structure of our society in any way?

Apart from highlighting concerns that are increasingly important for the whole of our society, this book describes a gripping emotional journey. It is testament to a remarkable woman with a wonderfully steadfast, loving and supportive family. Diane Blood, with her determination, love and courage, touched and enriched the lives of many people – many of whom she never even came into contact with. I am very glad that her important story can now be told and that I, in a very small way, was associated with it.

Robert Winston
London 2004

PROLOGUE

At 28 I had lived more than most. I had felt true love, happiness, hope, sorrow, grief, fear – a whole gamut of emotions that I cannot even begin to describe. I experienced them all in just one week – the week my husband died. On the Sunday morning of 26 February 1995, he had been a perfectly fit, healthy 30 year old, well enough to go to work. By that evening, he was too ill to communicate. Four days later, he was dead. I had watched him deteriorate through one of the most rapid and agonisingly painful diseases that one can possibly imagine.

People usually strive to describe death in comforting terms. When we pass on, we are supposed to just slip quietly away, but this pleasant piece of propaganda rarely holds out in truth. There was certainly nothing very serene about my husband's departure from this world, and I realise that this makes some uneasy. They said I should have let him die in peace, but this was never a possibility. It was not the fault of any medical procedure, but the ravages of the disease itself. Naturally, I was devastated. I don't like to see anyone suffer, but this was the man I would have gladly given my own life to save. By the evening of Thursday, 2 March, he was gone, but maybe I could still save our dreams.

By amazing coincidence, just a few months earlier we'd read about a widow who wished to have a baby by her deceased husband using his frozen semen. We commended her decision and concluded that, if we were ever in that situation, it was something that we would also wish to pursue. Against all the odds, it had been possible to extract some of my husband's sperm whilst he lay in a coma. My parents and my husband's family had all been consulted at the time. Everyone had agreed that the sperm should be taken, but it was also emphasised that no pressure would be put on me to go ahead with an attempted pregnancy if I later changed my mind.

11

For the next 18 months the possibility that I could still have my late husband's child was a closely kept family secret. I had no idea at the time of his death that this simple, private matter would subsequently lead to controversy and an extremely public High Court battle purely because I did not have his consent in writing.

In spite of losing my husband, I still considered myself very lucky, not just because our hope of a family was still alive but also because I was so incredibly grateful for the time we had shared together. I am painfully aware that some people never experience the warmth and intimacy of such a relationship. Perhaps that's why they didn't seem to have any true sympathy for how I felt. Many commented that I was lucky for entirely different reasons. They said that I was still young. That I'd find someone else.

The same had been said 12 years earlier when we'd first fallen in love. I was 16 years old. My husband had just turned 18. Young enough to be influenced by those who advised against rushing into anything, we'd waited over eight years before we married. Then the voices of authority had told me to study hard, to build a career before I started a family, to plan for the future and look ahead. Later I was to be questioned damningly for having done precisely that.

Forgive me if, given what I've been through, I am a little sceptical of other people's opinions. At times it seemed like I could not win, but I knew also that I could not lose. What I fought for was an issue of such central importance both to my life and to that of my late husband that my greatest loss would always have been to walk away. For that, I would never have forgiven myself. I even feared the enormous pressure on both my own and my husband's family might drive a wedge between us all that would have defeated what I had wanted to achieve. It would be no use winning the right to try for my husband's child if I lost the love and support of the caring extended family within which I had hoped to raise that child. This was just one of many seemingly impossible dilemmas I was to face. I wanted the rest of my life back. I fought for it at huge emotional and financial risk, but to have given in would have cost me my soul.

I am eternally grateful to all those who eased the burden along the way, to those who battled alongside me and, of course, to those who ultimately decided in my favour. In part, this story is a debt of gratitude to them. It is easy to say thank you, but the words mean very little without explaining the difference their actions made. I can't do it in a letter. Perhaps in a book I can get somewhere close.

To some, this may be a love story; to others, a nightmare – but for me, for the man I will always love, it is a plea that cold bureaucracy should never again be allowed to override raw human emotion.

I would like you to understand me and my late husband a little better. Perhaps by reading my story you can get beneath our skin, feel our blood flowing through your veins and begin to understand a little of what drives us and makes us who we are. We are all different. I recognise that the choices my late husband and I made may not be desirable to many, but this misses the point. You are not us. If you were, you would not question our wishes. If you were me, your heart would bleed as mine did. And you would ask that laws you'd always believed were set in stone, whether those of man or nature, be overturned.

CHAPTER 1

An ominous conversation

The phone rang. I was seized by a momentary rush of panic. There were deadlines to be met and still so much to do. It was a bit like the closing seconds of a school exam, when the teacher's voice first breaks the silence and you know your time is up. Mercifully, Tim, my colleague, answered quickly and the disturbing ringing stopped.

'Is t'other 'un there?' I could imagine my husband's cheery voice on the other end, even though I was out of earshot. The call came from the office downstairs. Stephen, or Steph (pronounced Steff) as I'd always known him, worked for my father's company in the same building as us, so his calls were a familiar ritual. He needed a lift home. Tim handed over the receiver on his way out the door, without ever having to explain who the caller was.

'Are we goin' 'ome tonight?'

'I'll not be long, I just want to finish off what I'm doing,' I remonstrated.

I hated home time, not because I disliked going home but because it meant that yet another day had passed in which I'd failed to achieve all that I'd hoped.

It had been two years since I'd set up Pseudonym Advertising. We had some tasty accounts and a portfolio of work which an agency ten times our size would be proud of, but there were still only two of us working there and time was ticking on. I'd ideally have liked to have taken on a few more employees before I contemplated starting a family, but we'd now been married for almost four years. Steph, who adored children, was beginning to get impatient and I, too, had started reading the agency's voucher copies of childcare magazines with more than just a professional interest. Finally recognising that life is never quite ideal, I'd given in to the constant requests and thrown away my diaphragm and half-finished tubes of spermicide. Now, a couple of months later with my period just overdue, I was more excited than Steph.

'Come upstairs and see me,' I invited. 'I'm waiting for the computer to print.'

Stephen plodded up the uncarpeted wooden stairs and plonked himself down on the chair beside the computer with the resigned air of one who knows that 'not long' could mean anything between five minutes and three hours but was more likely to be the latter.

'Has everyone else gone?'

He nodded, and for a second I caught a glimpse of weariness in his deep blue eyes.

'It'll not be long now, love, I promise.' I stepped one leg over his lap, sat on his knee facing him and began to gently kiss his forehead. I moved down to his eyes, closing them and kissing his long dark lashes as I went. 'It'll not be long until we have a family like everyone else and then I'll not work so hard, I promise.'

He smiled, hopefully, and squeezed my hand. I was so lucky to have such an understanding husband. At times I barely understood myself, but I had to be independent. I had lost my job four times. I'd been made redundant twice since we'd been married, so I felt the need to prove to myself that I could be successful. To be honest, I had finally started to believe in myself. We'd just produced our first agency brochure and Steph had been so proud of the finished result. It almost made it all seem worth it.

I glanced back at the computer. It was still barely halfway through processing the print information. I silenced Stephen's sighs by quickly moving my kisses down past his cheeks and onto his lips. As I absorbed his breath, I drew closer into him, wrapping my feet around the back legs of the chair and pulling myself tight against him so that in the heat of the moment we might melt into one.

The computer bleeped and for a second I was propelled back to reality. I leant back to press the return key, but Steph was hooked and caught hold of a few strands of my long fair hair, reeling me back towards him with a mischievous glint in his eyes.

I giggled like a nervous teenager. When you've been together for as long as we had, it is easy to allow familiarity to dull the edge, but in many ways our relationship was brand new. Trying for a family added fresh excitement.

The printer finally whirred into action. The spell was temporarily broken.

'Does that mean we can go now?'

'Yes,' I smiled.

We arrived home five minutes later and a good two and a half hours later than the average nine-to-five office worker. A quick look in the kitchen cupboards soon confirmed what I already knew. Last weekend had been one of the many when I hadn't had a chance to get to the supermarket.

'Do you fancy going for a pub meal?' I enquired, checking the cupboards for a second time, just to see if I could find anything more inspiring if I looked properly.

'Yeahhh,' Steph grinned enthusiastically, eager to avoid the wait even more than the washing up.

Luckily for Steph, I'd learnt not to be one of those women who take ages to get ready. I dashed into the bedroom and in a few seconds I made myself presentable.

We piled into the car and headed back down the road to our local. During the week, it served two two-course meals for a fiver, so eating out wasn't really an extravagance. Steph couldn't have enjoyed it if it was. He was always very cautious with money.

We quickly ordered our meals and sat down at the only dining table left – in a dimmed corner right next to the serving area. The smells drifted past temptingly as the waitresses flopped in and out of the kitchen with everyone else's meals. Thankfully it wasn't long before two large plates were placed on our table and we tucked in eagerly.

'Do you think we should tell my mum we're trying for a family?' I enquired.

'I think she already knows – or at least suspects. She doesn't miss a lot, your mam.'

'Maybe.'

'I think your parents'd love it if they had grandkids, although I don't think they'd cope too well running round after them.'

'No. I wish we were all a lot younger. Time just creeps up on you, doesn't it?'

17

'I was going to have paid off the mortgage and made my first million by the time I was 30,' sighed Steph wistfully.

'I know. But we're still doing better than most people our age.' It was a feeble attempt at cheering him up.

'Did I tell you I'd been to see the building society about our finances yesterday?' Steph leant forward slightly as the pace of his conversation quickened.

He had told me several times, but he continued before I could reply. 'We're five grand in front on our mortgage repayments.'

I smiled. I was so proud of him, mainly for being proud of himself. Trying to get rich never made him too busy to earn a living, and it was nice that he had something to show for all those years of cramming in the overtime. I leant over and squeezed his hand.

'Di,' he said, taking advantage of the moment of intimacy, 'is our marriage everything you hoped for?'

I pondered for a moment, not wanting to give a flippant answer. 'I'm happy enough, but I wish we'd married sooner. I think we missed a lot.'

Thankfully the sentiment didn't need further explanation. 'I do too in some ways. Do you know there was one point when I just couldn't get you out my mind, but I couldn't carry on like that. It was too intense. You'd burn yourself out.'

'I know. I used to feel like that too.' The memory brought a smile to my face.

I'd met my husband at a party or, to be more accurate, a series of parties, when I was still in the sixth form at school. It wasn't one of those grown-up type of introductions where you meet someone, get talking and find out you have a lot in common. In fact, I don't think we held a proper conversation until our first date. There was a definite magnetism, but initially it wasn't really to do with looks either. At least not on my part, and the first time we met, Steph had had so much to drink that I would have been surprised if he could see straight. Strictly speaking, we didn't even meet at the party, but at its exit. Steph had positioned himself just outside the door so he could collect a goodbye kiss from all the girls on their way home and beg them not to leave him. So that was our first kiss. A quick peck on the lips, which didn't really impress Steph. He couldn't even remember it. He was more taken with my friend, who gave him a nice big snog. But there was something about his eyes that I'd never forget.

An ominous conversation

It was his eyes I recognised when a mutual friend first introduced us a couple of months later at an organised bonfire and firework party. No fireworks for us, though, just a quick exchange of names and then we parted company. At least I remembered his name, which was more than could be said for him. He was never good with names, which was why he called everyone 'Duck'.

The next time we met was at another party just after Christmas. Steph was on a mission. One of those 'my mate fancies your mate' efforts. My friend wasn't interested and to be honest neither was I. This whole issue of teenage dating and the angst of who fancied who left me rather cold. I did envy those who genuinely seemed in love, but it always seemed to end in tears. A couple of guys asked me out that night. I declined. Steph asked for my phone number. I mumbled something about him being able to get it from the friend who'd introduced us at the bonfire and then left. I'd figured he'd never ask for it. He didn't. Still, at least I had something vaguely interesting to write about in my diary.

I wrote in it every night. It was probably no different from that of the average 16 year old. On most days, if I was being factually honest, it read something along the lines of 'Got up. Went to school. Walked home. Did my homework. Washed my hair. Went to bed.' Life, however hectic, can sound unbelievably banal when you commit it to paper. At times I got tired of writing the same old garbage, but I thought my diaries might be useful if I ever had a teenage daughter – just to remind me what it felt like – so I kept writing. It was a bit of a ritual and, besides, it was good practice. I wanted to be a writer when I left school.

I was especially annoyed at myself for not having anything very exciting to write on Valentine's Day. It's not that I didn't get any cards – just that I knew who they were from and I'd rather they hadn't bothered. Maybe it was time for me to fall in love, so I prayed that I would meet someone very special at the birthday party I was going to the evening after next. I prayed that this person would be so special that it would be the man I would eventually marry. I didn't want to go through all this heartache nonsense.

At the party on 16 February 1983, Steph asked me out. We didn't really spend the evening together. In fact, I think that one question was the sum total of our conversation. He asked if I would like to go out on the Saturday evening. I wasn't convinced he was the answer to my prayers, so I gave him my phone number on the tiniest scrap of paper you could possibly imagine and I deliberately didn't write my name. I was sure he'd never remember and I figured he'd need divine intervention not to lose a piece of paper so small before the weekend.

On Saturday, he called. I answered the phone, so he didn't need to know my name, which was fortunate for him because he later confessed to me that he had forgotten and wasn't quite sure how to ask for me if someone else had answered. I couldn't go out, as my parents were going out and I'd already invited my friend Helen round for a girls' night in. I suppose I could have changed my plans. Apparently he thought so too, but at the time he just suggested he'd call me the following night instead. I agreed. If this was the man I was destined to marry, I was sure he wouldn't let a little thing like my apparent indifference put him off. Later I learnt that it almost did, but something told him that he had to ring me, so, still without knowing my name, he called again on Sunday lunchtime.

Our first date was a Sunday afternoon stroll and that was when I fell in love. I couldn't believe I had been so careless as to almost miss this guy. We didn't part company until late that night. It felt as though we'd known each other for eternity. We talked endlessly. We walked for miles. And somewhere in those deep blue eyes I got hopelessly lost. They say that the eyes are the windows to the soul. Perhaps that was why Steph's eyes had haunted me since I'd first looked into them all those months ago. I was looking at my soulmate. We never looked back.

My prayer was answered. Our relationship stood the test of time and endured spending time apart when I went away to study copywriting at a college in London in 1984–5. We missed each other terribly at that time, even though I travelled home to Nottinghamshire most weekends.

We married on 11 May 1991. It was a big church wedding with all the trimmings. We used the traditional Anglican 1662 Book of Common Prayer service. Steph insisted. It placed greater emphasis on procreation and meant I had to answer that I would 'obey' him. Most brides preferred the more modern version because it omitted that particular phrase and didn't place so much importance on raising children. I happily agreed with Steph.

He looked so handsome and wore a big grin as I walked up the aisle to join him. Afterwards, we held a reception in a marquee on the lawn of my parents' bungalow. It was very pretty, draped in peach, with pale blue and peach flowers hanging from the poles and decorating each table. In the evening we had a disco. Our first dance was to 'Endless Love'. Weddings pass so quickly, but a friend gave me a good piece of advice, 'Take time out to be alone and tell each other how special the day is, even if it is only for a few seconds.'

Steph and I sneaked around the back of the marquee. We held hands, looked at one another and soaked up the atmosphere of the occasion. I treasure those few moments we spent together away from our guests, but it was also nice to be able to share our happiness with friends and family. It couldn't have been more perfect. Now all we had to do was make the rest of our dreams come true.

We had let almost four years pass us by. They were comfortable years, despite the upheavals with my career. Steph had changed jobs, too. He left the galvanising company, where he had worked ever since I met him, and began working for my father's kitchen and bathroom installation company shortly after our marriage. Even so, I think that Steph, in particular, having just turned 30 a couple of weeks before, was beginning to suffer an early mid-life crisis. We wanted more out of life and we were looking forward to the excitement and challenges of raising a family. It was time to move on with our plans.

The sound of Steph's voice brought me back to the present. 'Do you know, there was so much I wanted to achieve in my life and there's so little time to do it?'

'I know, I feel like I'm getting old too.'

'You should write that book you used to go on about.'

'No, I haven't experienced enough to write about. Besides, I'm happy writing advertisements. It's more fun.'

'That's it, you see, at least you've got your company. If I died, I'd want to be remembered for something. I'd want the name "Blood" to go down in history, to have invented something or been the first to do something, to have contributed – made the world a better place.'

'When we have kids, you'll be remembered by them. That's all most people get,' I ventured.

'I know, and I know they'd have the family name, but I want

more than most people. When I die, I'd hope to have a church full of people all saying what a great guy I was.'

'You are a great guy. Does it matter what anyone thinks or says when you're dead?'

The question remained unanswered. Instead he pondered for a moment. 'What would you do if owt ever 'appened to me? Could you cope now?' He took it for granted that, like him, during that earlier intensity in our relationship the pain of losing him would have been too much to even contemplate, let alone bear.

Even so, the thought still stabbed at my heart. A brief frown flickered across my forehead. 'Yes, I think I'd survive – I wouldn't remarry, though. There'd be no point.'

'No, I wouldn't either if owt happened to you. What would you do? Would you keep the house?'

I swallowed hard. We'd worked hard on our bungalow, taking three years to lovingly do it all up before we married and moved in. 'Yes. I'd carry on.'

Steph nodded his approval.

Thankfully, the waitress arrived with the sweets and the conversation ended. It was becoming too painful for both of us. We ate our dessert in silence.

'Ready?' Steph tried to strike a more cheery note as I swallowed my last mouthful. Without having to give a verbal response, I picked up the car keys and led the way out into the cold, still night air.

The car park was flanked by open fields and was lit by a single white streetlight to whose feeble warmth the mist clung for dear life. On this dank February evening, every breath hung in the air and every utterance left its trail. We walked quickly for fear the words we had exchanged would stay with us forever.

Little did I realise that by the same time next week my husband would be dead.

CHAPTER 2

Stephen becomes unwell

The weekend Steph fell terminally ill began inconspicuously enough. I awoke on Saturday morning to the sensation of gentle kisses being planted on my naked skin. Steph had obviously been awake for some time and was bored. As soon as I opened my eyes, he stopped and grinned, looking rather pleased with himself. I didn't like being woken up, but he knew that this way I couldn't be mad at him.

'It's your turn to make coffee.'

'No,' I moaned. 'You were awake first, you should bring me a drink.'

'I make it all week. It's only fair you make it at weekends.'

It was an argument I couldn't win, so I promised to make it when I'd had time to come to. I turned over and snuggled back down to catch a few precious extra seconds of relaxation.

The peace was broken. 'A few seconds is up.'

'No-o-o.'

'Ye-e-es.'

It was in danger of turning into the familiar pantomime we played every weekend. *Oh, no it isn't – oh, yes it is*. So this time I decided to give in gracefully and go and make the coffee. Besides, today I had reason to get up. He'd promised we could go and fetch the last bedroom unit for the spare bedroom he'd been fitting out. We needed more storage space for when we had our baby. It wasn't really nursery furniture, but we'd picked it because we thought it would look nice in a kid's bedroom. I reminded Steph about going to fetch the unit, whilst wafting the coffee teasingly under his nose. Bribery seemed as good a way as any to ensure he hadn't changed his mind.

We were soon on our way to the furniture store. It was a good half-hour journey, so we passed the time cheerfully discussing our favourite topic of the moment: babies. No, Steph would prefer not to be present at the birth. No, he didn't think he'd want to know the baby's sex before it was born. He'd probably prefer a girl, but a son would be nice too.

Names? Well, we'd chosen the name if it was a girl. We'd decided on Shannon. Steph had first suggested the name. We'd enjoyed a few precious days' break in Limerick when we'd attended my cousin's wedding last summer, and he claimed to have been influenced by the beautiful Shannon River. I rather thought he'd been more influenced by the beautiful Nicole Kidman who played Shannon in *Far and Away*, a film we'd recently watched together on TV, but what the heck, it was a nice-sounding name – and I had enjoyed the film too.

We arrived at the retail park and went in to fetch the unit. It took a while to arrive at the collection point, so I waited for it while Steph popped into Texas Homecare, which was next door. My father's company, where Steph worked, organised their kitchen and bathroom installations. Steph wanted to call in and see someone while he was there. Like me, he was always working even on his days off.

Eventually the unit arrived and I happily scrawled my signature across the bottom of the paperwork. It still gave me a thrill to sign my husband's surname, even though we'd been married for nearly four years. As the company I was working for went into receivership whilst I was on honeymoon and I needed to rely on my former reputation for freelance assignments, I'd chosen to stick to my maiden name for work. Somehow that made it even more special when I could use my married name.

On the way home we considered going to Sheffield to do a spot of clothes shopping. Steph needed some new stuff for work, but I moaned that I needed to get some work done. The decision to leave the shopping expedition till next week was swayed by the fact that Steph also felt a bit under the weather. We went home.

The folder and leaflet I was working on took most of the

weekend to write, although I did allow myself a break to watch a film on TV with Steph on the Saturday evening. We thought Steph must be coming down with flu because his limbs ached and he felt pretty lousy, but he didn't have the accompanying sniffles. I teased that I thought it was really an excuse to get him out of fitting the bedroom. It was a long-standing joke that my husband was very good at starting jobs but always seemed to lose interest when they were 95 per cent complete. The problem was, he always had to do everything himself. No one else came up to his exacting standards. There was another reason too. He was proud that, in years to come, he'd be able to stand back and say, 'I did that!', and he looked forward to the day he could tell our children. We liked our home and didn't plan on moving, so he even had plans to extend.

On Saturday night, we went to bed at the usual time. Steph seemed very hot. I thought he must have a temperature and I was a bit concerned. Perhaps he'd be better in the morning.

I woke reasonably early on Sunday morning and resolved to go and make the coffee without a fight. I turned over and my heart leapt into my mouth. I fervently patted the empty space at the side of me. Nothing. Steph never got up without waking me first.

'Steph, Steph,' I cried at the top of my voice.

'It's OK, I'm here.' His voice was encouragingly calm as he walked into the bedroom.

'Oh-h,' I sank back into the pillow, as the pounding in my heart slowed to its usual rhythm. 'I didn't know where you were. I was worried you'd gone.'

'I couldn't sleep, so I got up early,' he explained. 'I've got to go and meet someone at work in a few minutes. They're coming to collect a bathroom and I said I'd be there.'

'Oh. Will you be long?'

'No, I shouldn't be.'

I relaxed. How stupid of me to panic. I hated not knowing where he was. That's what was so reassuring about being married. No matter what he'd been doing or what the day brought, each evening he was there lying by my side and I knew he was safe.

When we were first courting, Steph had a motorbike. We lived a couple of miles apart and it was useful as he could get up and see me easily, but whenever he was late or if he'd been out for a ride, my nerves were on edge until he called or I heard the delightful roar of the 250cc engine as it mounted the little hill into our drive.

I'd been relieved when he'd finally got rid of it. Not because I didn't like motorbikes. If I'd been riding pillion, I wouldn't have worried in the slightest – at least if anything happened we'd have been together – but he'd had more than his fair share of accidents and every time I feared the worst. Once he'd fallen off and dislocated his shoulder. He'd had to be taken to hospital so his sister called me to explain why he hadn't arrived to see me when he was supposed to. I'd almost worn the carpet out pacing up and down all afternoon, and when the phone finally rang, I could have cried with sheer relief that someone knew where he was. He was injured, but at least he was safe.

After all these years knowing that disaster didn't strike at every turn, I was learning to be less paranoid, but I would still have the occasional panic. I'd once temporarily lost Stephen on a beach. He'd been for a swim and had lost his bearings when he'd returned to the shore. He was missing for ages and I'd really started to worry for his safety. When he eventually found me, I was so relieved, but I also felt slightly foolish that I had panicked so much.

By the time Steph returned from work, I'd almost finished writing the leaflets. He sat quietly on the settee and said he was feeling a little better. I made some dinner, an abridged version of the usual mammoth Sunday lunch (without the Yorkshire puddings). Steph made a valiant attempt to eat it and complimented my cooking. He wished he'd been able to enjoy it more. After clearing up, it was my turn to go to work.

'I want to go in and typeset this copy, so it's all done and out of the way for Monday morning. I've got three ads to write, too, so if I get this done it'll be one less to worry about. I shouldn't be long.'

The famous last words. We both knew everything always took longer than I expected, but Steph encouraged me to go and get it over with. He knew I wouldn't rest, leaving the job only half done.

It could be quite lonely at work, upstairs in my little office, so I was happy when I heard my father's footsteps enter the building. Besides, I'd almost finished and it meant I wouldn't have to lock up on my own, a tedious process at the best of times but even more annoying after a hard weekend's slog, when all you wanted to do was get home for a nice relaxing evening.

'Dad?'

'Yeah,' came the confirmation.

'Oh, hi. I was just about to go home.'

'Stephen rang your mum. He's feeling worse and he wanted to know if she knew where he could get any antibiotics. I'll bring the thermometer and come up and have a look at him later.'

I left immediately and in reality my dad arrived at my house only a few minutes behind me. Steph's temperature was a little high, so, after my father had left, I tried to cool him down with a cold flannel.

'I don't know, fancy going and getting sick, especially when it's been such a lovely sunny day.' I was talking rubbish, as if being ill was somehow easier if it was slinging it down with rain. 'Don't go and give it to me. I don't want your germs.'

'I tell you what, Di,' Steph responded after some delay, 'I really do hope you don't get this. It's terrible.'

I continued to apply the cold flannel to his now boiling forehead. 'There, does that feel any better?' I soothed, kneeling down beside him.

'No.'

I obviously wasn't doing it right, so I got some more cold water and tried again. I took his temperature. It was higher. More cold water. Still he felt worse. I was doing my best. Why wasn't it working? Perhaps the big electric fan from work would help. I phoned my dad to say I was going to fetch it, but he volunteered to go instead. He dropped it off shortly afterwards, just in time to empty the bucket which Stephen had filled with vomit a few minutes earlier, which was fortunate as I am very squeamish.

I'd tried to get him to clean it up himself, but he'd looked at me with big pitiful eyes. 'Di, I can't. I'm too ill.'

I couldn't deal with it, as I knew that if I caught the smell, I'd join in.

Once again we were left alone, the fan positioned on the table at one end of the settee, the sick bucket at the other and Stephen laid out between them, complaining that I was trying to freeze him to death with the fan. He wouldn't believe me that he was really hot and fought like hell when I tried to take his T-shirt off. He was so annoyed, he decided to go to bed. Good. I could turn the radiator off in the room, put the fan on, shut the door and let him rest. I couldn't understand why his temperature wasn't coming down. I was shivering like mad.

I soon warmed up, but I couldn't relax. I was in and out of the room like a yo-yo. He kept turning the fan off and pleaded with me not to turn it on again. I called the doctor, who confirmed he probably had flu and I was doing the right thing, although he said that he had to come out later anyway, so he would call round before going to bed.

I tried writing my advertisements. I made some herbal tea. I turned the fan back on and made some more herbal tea, but I didn't drink it. I went back into the room and cradled Stephen in my arms as he was sick once again. Strangely enough, the smell of regurgitated dinner festering in the bucket no longer bothered me, and I was quite proud of myself for coping. I wondered if that's what would happen when we had kids. It often amazed me how friends who had been just as squeamish as me never even flinched when having to deal with their children's smelly mess. When someone we love cannot help themselves, maybe that's what happens, I thought – we just get on with doing what has to be done.

'It'll be all right. You'll be OK.'

Stephen no longer responded. Where was that doctor?

Eventually my impatience was rewarded and a torch light flashed past the kitchen window. We didn't have a number on the house, so I knew the search was fruitless. I ran a few paces down the drive and then remembered to walk.

I sounded quite collected as I enquired, 'Are you the doctor?', and directed him to the bedroom.

'Stephen, sit up. The doctor's here to see you.' I tried to sound authoritative and was embarrassed by his lack of cooperation.

'Does that hurt?' the doctor asked as he tried to straighten Stephen's legs.

'Aaah-ah-ah,' was the only response we could get.

'I think that means it hurts,' I translated. 'He's not usually like this. He's not a bad patient. He doesn't normally complain.'

'Can you try and bend your head?' the doctor asked.

No response.

The doctor tried again in a louder voice, 'Can you get your chin to touch your chest?' He forced Stephen's head forwards.

This time I also winced with pain. 'You're hurting him.'

'It's probably flu,' the doctor pronounced. 'A temperature can cause those kind of reactions, but I think we'd better have him in hospital – just to be sure.'

'What else could it be?'

'Well, there's a slim chance it could be meningitis.'

I'd heard of meningitis and knew that it was something to do with the brain. I also knew that it was a serious disease but had thought that it normally affected small children. I didn't really understand the implications of what the doctor had said. I wanted to ask more, but we were still in the bedroom and I didn't want my questions to frighten Stephen. I didn't know if he could hear or not.

I'd vaguely imagined that I would have to drive him to the hospital, but the doctor went into the lounge to use the phone to book him into the ward and call the ambulance. No, it wasn't that urgent, but an ambulance some time in the next half-hour would be nice. The doctor left. I called my parents, who lived only two minutes away. My father came straight away, whilst my mother packed some toiletries. The ambulance arrived before him.

'I don't know how you're going to get him into the ambulance. He's not being too cooperative.'

'We'll manage,' the two ambulance men reassured me.

They quickly decided that our home had too many tight corners for a stretcher and settled on a chair lift.

I coaxed Stephen into a sitting position on the edge of the bed. The ambulance men needed me to hold the doors open, but Stephen needed me more. He was sick again. I held my arms around him and he rested his head on my shoulder. I needed him too. The heat from his body radiated into mine and something more, something very precious but hard to explain. From that moment, I knew I was on my own – the guardian of our hopes, dreams and ambitions. Steph had always been the strong one, but now he was no longer capable of helping himself. I had to make decisions and do everything for him.

Despite the lack of my assistance, the ambulance men clattered into the bedroom and the moment of intimacy was broken. I dressed Steph in his dressing gown and some slippers and somehow he gathered enough strength to make it from the edge of the bed to the chair. They carried him into the ambulance and laid him down.

My father arrived in time to lock up and follow the ambulance in his car. I went with Stephen.

He groaned a little as the engine started up.

'I think he's still feeling sick. Perhaps if you had a container?'

The ambulance man reached up, grabbed a suitable receptacle

and held it at Stephen's side. The groaning stopped. Deathly silence.

'Stephen. Stephen?'

There was the roar of the engine changing gear and – nothing, absolutely no human sound whatsoever. Not a breath from anyone, nor the faintest beat of a heart.

The ambulance man continued, shaking Stephen's arm slightly as he raised his voice, 'Stephen, are you all right?'

After a split second, which seemed to last a lifetime, Steph grunted.

We'd held our breath for so long that we exhaled in bursts, almost laughing. How silly of us to panic.

'I bet you're worried sick, aren't you?' The ambulance man turned towards me as he spoke.

I didn't answer. I was concentrating on my husband's body, which was rocking helplessly to and fro as we trundled down the street.

'Don't worry. He'll be all right. He's going to the best place.'

I hoped he meant the hospital.

I felt terribly alone as we rolled up the hospital corridors and into the lift to the ward. If the emotional solitude was too much to bear, our physical parting was to be even more traumatic. My father and I were apprehended at the ward door. The trolley rolled on. I clung to its sides, until my arm could stretch no further. We were torn apart. I felt as though my heart had been ripped from my body.

'Please. I want . . .'

The nurse interrupted, 'We have to get him settled into bed. Then you can see him. You can wait in the day room.'

The nurse directed us to the little room off the side of the corridor. She sounded so calm. They were going to get him 'settled'. Perhaps all was well after all. I shouldn't worry so much.

My mother joined us in the day room. She'd packed the essential toiletries and some pyjamas. (My husband didn't possess any, so I'd sent him to hospital dressed only in his boxer shorts and dressing gown.) I was amazed she'd managed to find us, but I shouldn't have been.

My mother was a lot tougher than anyone gave her credit for and could usually be relied upon in a crisis. If there had been a kettle in the room she'd have been making the tea, but there were no such home comforts, just rows and rows of hard metal-framed chairs, an old TV, which might have broken the silence during the day, and a large clock, with a dedication to someone, ticking away slowly and loudly on the wall.

A doctor appeared – a lady. No, a girl really. She looked younger than me. I expected her to reassure me that Stephen was settled and stable, but if I was waiting for a calm, comforting voice I was to be disappointed. She sounded as anxious as I was, which was really quite unnerving. We are conditioned to expect doctors to at least pretend everything is under control even when it isn't, so I knew things must be pretty bad. Perhaps it was her inexperience that gave so much away, but in many ways I was grateful, not only because I couldn't stand being patronised but also because at least I knew they were concerned enough to treat the case with the urgency it deserved.

'Is your husband normally aggressive?' she asked.

What a strange question, I thought. 'No, not really. Why?'

'Well, he's reacting quite violently.'

'He didn't want me to help him earlier and he was a bit angry when I kept turning the cold fan on him, but I wouldn't say he was aggressive.'

I looked to my parents to substantiate my claim. They agreed.

The doctor looked increasingly concerned. 'I don't quite know how to say this, but it's a question I have to ask. Could he have taken drugs?'

'I gave him some Day Nurse earlier.' I paused, puzzled. I got the impression she wasn't talking about 20 ml of cold remedy. Then I immediately started wondering if he'd taken more. Yes that was it! The Day Nurse. When I'd given him the measure before I went to work, the bottle had been quite full. When I came home, I was sure it was nearly empty and he'd probably also taken paracetamol.

I conveyed my fears to the doctor. She didn't seem to think it was significant, but by now I was convinced. There had to be some logical explanation. My poor husband, he'd been in so much pain, he'd accidentally taken an overdose, rather than complain too loudly.

The doctor went back to see her patient and I duly dispatched my mother to fetch the Day Nurse bottle. It turned out to be a waste of time. It wasn't the Day Nurse.

A short while later, the doctor appeared again. More questions, but no real answers. Yes, Steph had had a lot of illnesses recently. He'd had a lot of colds. Yes, he had had a strange rash, but it was about six months ago and had been diagnosed as an allergic reaction. Yes, he'd recently developed an allergy to feather pillows. I didn't think I could be of any more help, but apparently I might. They were trying to shine light into his eyes to check the reaction, but he wouldn't keep them open and they wanted me to see if I could persuade him to be a little more cooperative. I was pleased to be allowed in the room to see him. My father suggested Stephen might respond better to his more authoritative approach, but they'd only let one of us in the room, so it was down to me.

When I walked into the room, there were crowds of people round his bed and I was shocked at how much his condition seemed to have deteriorated. I'd left him in their care and it was going wrong. I wanted to take him back into my arms, send them all away and care for him myself, but I knew I couldn't. He seemed so unapproachable lying there with all these strangers around him. He was fighting like hell and swearing at anyone who touched him. It wasn't like my husband, and when all the medical staff had failed to make him see sense and open his eyes, how was I supposed to make him respond to me, just because I was his wife, in a situation that was anything but intimate?

'Stephen, it's me, Diane. Can you hear me?'

I was ushered to the top of the bed.

He stopped thrashing and swearing, but I think that had more to do with everyone else temporarily stopping prodding him than any reaction to my voice.

'Stephen, it's all right. I'm here. You've got to open your eyes so they can make you better.'

There was no response, so I gently pulled open one of his lids. Success! The doctor shone the light in and managed to get quite a good look without him fighting or pulling away. I'd managed to do what no one else had been able to do, but the sense of achievement was short lived. Stephen had obviously decided that he'd put up with enough pain and any attempt to repeat the performance with the other eye was not on. I lifted the lid a couple of times but couldn't hold it open for more than a few seconds. The doctor decided that perhaps she'd seen enough and gave up gracefully. I was sent back to the day room. She followed almost immediately behind me, preventing the need to relay the story to my parents twice.

They wanted to do a lumbar puncture and the senior doctor was on his way over. I was pleased. I thought he might have a few more answers.

The senior doctor arrived, introduced himself and assumed control. He told us about the lumbar puncture they were going to do. They would put a needle in Stephen's spine and extract some fluid to analyse.

He left to perform the task. Minutes later, he arrived back.

'We're having difficulty getting Stephen to lie still enough for us to do a lumbar puncture. Apparently, you managed to get him to open his eyes before. Perhaps you could get him to lie still?' He was addressing me.

Ah, so he wasn't in control after all. I trundled back into the room, somewhat deflated.

They needed Stephen to lie in the foetal position. I could get him into the right position, but he kicked out as soon as they touched him, screaming in pain. It was unbearable to hear. I asked for them to fetch my dad and the younger female doctor explained how my father had thought Stephen might listen to him.

I actually knew that Stephen was well past listening to anyone, but I needed the moral support in there. I was so frustrated that the doctors couldn't get what they needed, I thought that if we got enough men in the room maybe they could physically restrain Stephen.

My father was brought in but, after another couple of attempts, the mission was aborted. The doctor explained that it would be very dangerous if Stephen moved while the needle was in his spine. He didn't need to explain further. If it was obviously so risky, why had they persisted trying for so long? Even if they had managed to get the needle in, a blind man could see there was no way anyone could have kept him still.

I was glad that, for now, that particular danger was over and they could let Stephen rest, but at the same time I was pretty gutted they hadn't been able to get what they needed to find out what was wrong. I was frustrated with Stephen for not keeping still and getting it over with and even more annoyed at the doctors for not volunteering to come back for another attempt in a few hours. Everyone just seemed to expect me to accept that it was bed time, so nothing else could be done until the morning.

They put Stephen onto some antibiotics (which is how they said

33

they would treat him for meningitis anyway), hooked him up to a drip, said we could stay in the room and walked off leaving us in charge of keeping the drip dripping until the morning.

I was mentally exhausted and tried hard not to think too much. Steph had always told me that was one of my faults. Whenever I had previously worried, whether it was about Steph's safety or something less significant, it had always turned out fine in the end. We would come through this too. I just had to live through this awful period, project ourselves into the light at the other end of the tunnel and concentrate on getting there.

CHAPTER 3

Praying things will improve

The first half of the night passed too quickly. Before settling down, Steph had been thrashing about so much that the nurses had had to put cot sides up onto his bed. I was relieved when he finally rested, but then I was anxious because of his lack of movement. Occasionally, he turned his head. His eyes were open. I swapped sides, trying to connect with his blank stare, but the eyes that had always haunted me revealed nothing. A couple of times the drip stopped. One flick of the tube and it started again.

Gradually, as it got closer to morning, time began to drag. I was waiting for the doctor to come back and for Stephen's parents to arrive. They had only just returned from a holiday the day previously so had decided (as there was nothing they could really do to help the situation) not to come into the hospital until they heard how Steph was in the morning. My parents had tried to describe how ill he was, but I don't think they had any real comprehension of the situation until they saw him for themselves. It was so hard to imagine how someone could deteriorate so quickly. I had been sure that things would improve when everyone arrived. I felt there must be someone who could make it all better, but alas no. Stephen's parents were as helpless and dismayed as I was and the doctor had no magic wand either. There wasn't much anyone could do.

In the morning, they decided to introduce barrier nursing to avoid any spread of infection, so we all had to wear surgical masks and gloves. It must have looked incredibly intimidating. As people began prodding him again, Steph became increasingly agitated. He wanted to get up. He cursed and swore and fought everyone who stood in his way. He tried to communicate, but couldn't. At one point he said, 'Gotta go to work.' I reassured him that we were all having the day off and he temporarily relaxed, but something else was bothering him. I think he wanted to go to the loo, but no one would let him get out of bed and it was hardly surprising that he couldn't go when surrounded by all these people. It was a scene which during my later court ordeal was to flash through my mind so many times when my critics said I should have let my husband die in peace and dignity. Whichever way you gloss over it, there is nothing dignified about dying of meningitis. I could have done nothing to alter that. As for peace, it seems to me that life is not a terribly peaceful business. We come into this world screaming and my husband went out the same way. He was not one to lie down quietly and give in. I would not have expected him to.

It was decided to move Steph to a hospital in the neighbouring town of Mansfield so they could do a brain scan. They didn't particularly want to move him, but it was apparently essential. I was extremely frustrated that our local hospital didn't have the necessary equipment. They went to make the arrangements for the transfer and, on their return, they informed us that there had been a change of plan. They were now taking him to the Sheffield Hallamshire. They had sorted out the team who was to travel in the ambulance with my husband. We were to follow by car. I was unhappy about this and insisted on travelling in the ambulance. Reluctantly, they consented.

So that was it, we set off. A sad little convoy. My husband, the medical team and myself in the ambulance. Our parents following by car. I think I held my breath for most of the journey. The ambulance men wanted to know which was most important, speed or a smooth ride. The answer, of course, was both. The route to Sheffield was familiar enough. I'd travelled it many times, but I'd never realised before the number of lumps and bumps in the road. For most of the journey, we travelled in silence, but occasionally we 'blue lighted' through some traffic lights or an area where it was slightly more congested. How many times have we all heard that familiar ambulance siren and wondered about the fate of those it was attempting to help? I'd never imagined that I would be travelling in one.

On arrival at the Hallamshire, Steph was taken to the Admissions ward, a small room with around eight trolley beds and a desk. We were put at the end nearest the window. The medical staff who'd travelled with us sorted out the paperwork at the desk and then left.

Steph still wanted to go to the loo, at least that was my interpretation of the situation. He wanted to be up and off. Unfortunately, we now had a bed with no cot sides, so I was having a difficult job pinning him down. He kicked, cursed and bit. I shouted for help, but no one came. The bed didn't have its brakes on, so I'd wedged it up against the wall on one side and was managing to block the other with my body. The only route open to Steph was to go off the bottom of the bed. In a valiant attempt to escape, he managed to stand bolt upright on the bed. I tried to push him back down, but the bed wheeled precariously away from the wall and I was frightened he'd fall. The woman in the next bed must have been horrified by the whole pantomime. She was clutching an oxygen mask to help her breathe. She tried joining in my shouts for help. Her voice was very weak and under normal circumstances I would not have allowed her to continue shouting when she was obviously so ill herself. These were not normal circumstances, however, and I was grateful for her help.

The cavalry arrived. First a doctor from Neurology and then our families, who'd been dumped in a waiting room and had finally decided to go looking for someone who might be able to throw some light on our whereabouts. They didn't find anyone who could help, but they did find the Admissions ward. The whole thing was a total shambles. Until the moment that neurologist arrived, the Hallamshire seemed totally unprepared for the urgency and seriousness of the situation. In fairness to them, it seemed we'd been accidentally dumped on them with no medical notes. They had to ask the Bassetlaw to send them on by taxi. There had apparently been an argument about the health service not being reponsible for paying for this, until someone had been firm enough to point out that it was a matter of life and death.

Thankfully, from the moment the neurologist arrived I felt we were in good, capable hands. Despite the initial hiccup, for which I can only blame the exceptional circumstances of such a terrible illness, the Hallamshire did everything possible to save my husband's life.

There were more questions about drugs, trips abroad and the details of our sex life. They didn't pull any punches. They wanted as much information in as short a time as possible.

My answer was as blunt as their questioning. 'Why, do you think he has Aids?'

The doctor looked sheepish. 'No, it's just a young man, so very ill – we have to ask. It's routine with someone of this age.'

It wasn't routine to me. I think sex education lessons have got a bit more realistic these days, but when I was growing up we worried it might be possible to get pregnant just by touching and thought that sexually transmitted diseases were caught by sitting on toilet seats. No matter how ridiculous the question might have sounded, I was frightened. The media has taught the average adult to be afraid of HIV, but, at that time, nobody ever mentioned any risk of dying of meningitis. My feelings obviously didn't matter. My husband's life was at stake.

We were both strictly heterosexual. We'd been together for 12 years. We married in 1991 and we were trying for a baby. He'd been abroad once without me. He'd gone to Portugal to fit a kitchen. I'd bet my life that he'd never been unfaithful. He didn't do drugs (I could answer this one now I'd sorted out that they didn't mean the cold remedy) and, apart from the new tendency to curse, kick and bite when he was too ill to communicate by any other method, he didn't have any other nasty habits I thought the doctor should know about.

He looked relieved. Meningitis is rarely linked to HIV and, from what I'd said, he thought it an unlikely added complication.

Now we needed to do that brain scan, but, as with the lumbar puncture, we were to be defeated. Steph was in too much pain to cooperate and to do the scan he needed to lie still. The doctors made several attempts, but eventually the mission was abandoned. After almost a full day of following the bed around the hospital as Steph was wheeled from one place to another, he was finally admitted to his own little room on the Communicative Diseases ward and the barrier nursing sign was put up on the door.

We were shown into a smoke-filled day room. Some of its inhabitants tried to make small talk, which I wasn't in the mood for. I ran out to the toilet. I needed to go and throw up. By the time

I returned, the nursing staff had sorted out a separate room which was designed for relatives who wanted to sleep over w. their loved ones were ill. The room was a godsend. I don't kno. how the five of us would have coped if we hadn't had such a bolt hole.

I lost track of time. Day and night merged into one. In these situations someone always takes it upon themselves to try and focus your mind on normal routine. In this case, it was my dad. 'You need to eat . . . You need to sleep . . . You really ought to go home, change your clothes and get a wash.'

He thought it'd make me feel better. How ridiculous can you get? Getting changed would hardly alter my husband's critical state. Besides, I might miss something important and I didn't think the world would collapse if I temporarily forgot about my personal hygiene. I wasn't going anywhere, but the night without sleep combined with the general worry was beginning to lead to emotional exhaustion.

I was with Stephen's parents in his room when a doctor came in to administer some drugs to prevent me from catching meningitis. He asked if I was taking the pill, as it would be affected by what he was about to prescribe. I confirmed that I wasn't but had to add that we were trying for a family and there was a chance I could be pregnant. I thought back to our conversation in the pub before Stephen became ill. Should we tell my parents we were trying? We hadn't even discussed whether to tell his parents. This certainly wasn't how I'd wanted to announce it to them. I'd planned to arrive at their house one day all smiles and carrying a little pair of woollen booties.

The doctor had to go off and check whether I could still take the tablets if I was pregnant. He came back a few minutes later and said I could. Tablets were also prescribed for my father. As we were the ones who had spent the evening with Steph before barrier nursing was introduced, we were those perceived to be most at risk.

Later that evening it was finally possible for the doctors to carry out a brain scan. Steph had calmed down somewhat after eventually peeing himself and being fitted with a catheter to avoid the problem recurring – a further mockery of the notion of 'death with dignity'. They had actually hoped for a couple of different brain scans, but they could only get one before Steph became too agitated again. For once, it was good news. There were no signs of swelling around the brain. When he recovered, he wouldn't be left brain damaged. It was the first time anyone had said 'when' he recovered. I had previously feared that 'if' might have been a more accurate word.

In general, meningitis proves fatal in 10 per cent of cases, but I wasn't really given any information about Steph's particular chances of overcoming the disease and I didn't ask. There wasn't time, everything was too intense. I needed the doctors to concentrate their energies on making my husband better, not sharing their knowledge with me. We were focusing on each little step rather than worrying about the overall picture. After hearing the good news from the scan, we were even quite jovial. Speaking metaphorically, my dad said that I'd just won the lottery. I really felt as though I had.

That night I grabbed a couple of hours of disturbed shut-eye in between keeping a bedside vigil in Stephen's room with his mother. Everyone said he seemed to be improving, but I couldn't see it. In fact, I thought his condition was deteriorating.

The next morning, the mission to get me to go home continued. I was having none of it, although my dad did manage to persuade Stephen's mum to go home for a brief while. He drove her while my mum and Stephen's dad stayed at the hospital with me.

Today, the lumbar puncture was back on the agenda. Stephen was no more likely to stay still now than before. I was becoming increasingly emotionally worn down with each mini battle. He was not going to be brain damaged, but paralysis caused by a lumbar puncture gone wrong was not something my husband could have survived and coped with. He had tremendous admiration for the disabled, but if it was to happen to him, he always reckoned death would be preferable.

Doctors in a busy hospital are under severe time constraints. I was the one who had spent most of the night watching my husband, not them. I didn't want them just to launch in and do a lumbar puncture without realising how much he would fight. They thought it would be OK. I didn't. Stephen's dad backed me up. They went in to see Steph, prodded him a couple of times and decided that perhaps we were right.

For now, at least, it was the end of another immediate danger, but I was becoming increasingly restless. They were only gone for a couple of hours, but I couldn't wait for my dad and Stephen's mum to return. In my opinion, Steph was deteriorating rapidly and I thought that when they came back it would make it all better. Something had to. Besides which, the doctors would be back to see about the lumbar puncture again later and I was about done in. I wasn't up for yet another battle, having to explain that Steph wouldn't keep still. I needed their support.

In the event, there were no more disagreements about the lumbar puncture. By the time the doctors returned again that afternoon, Steph's condition had altered. He seemed to be in a deep sleep, quite still and calm. It was as safe as it was ever going to be to carry out the procedure. Apart from the danger of sudden movement leading to paralysis, I also knew that the trauma created by a lumbar puncture could cause other serious complications. I hadn't missed the fact that the cardiac massage machine had been waiting outside my husband's room ever since he had been admitted. It was a risky time and I wanted to be with him just in case. The doctors wanted me out of the way. We came to a compromise. I could stay in the room and hold Stephen's hand as long as I didn't get in their way if anything went wrong.

Thankfully the whole thing went very smoothly. Now they could analyse the spinal fluid and hopefully get some answers. I felt as though I'd just run a marathon but then some swine had gone and moved the finishing line. I wanted to rest, but it wasn't over yet.

Stephen's mum and dad returned to their post by his bedside. I wandered back and forth between his room and our little bolt hole. I knew they'd call me if anything dramatic happened. The only thing they had to report was that he had started to snore, which I could hear for myself. In all the time I'd known my husband, he'd never once snored. I thought he couldn't breathe and I went to fetch the male nurse. He put something on my husband's finger to check the oxygen level in his blood. It was fine.

My parents were resting in our room, Steph's parents were watching over him in his, and I was wearing out my shoe leather trekking between the two. The aggravated breathing was getting worse each time I returned. I wanted to fetch the nurse again but didn't want to keep troubling him unnecessarily. I consulted Steph's mum and dad, but they thought he was just snoring. I couldn't take it any more. I had to get out. I went to ask my dad to go in and see what he thought. My dad was exhausted too, but after taking a minute to compose himself he obediently trotted down the corridor to have a look.

Seconds later he flew back in through the door of our room in tears, with Stephen's parents following hot on his heels.

'Cardiac arrest,' he blurted. 'As I got to the door they shouted, "Cardiac arrest".'

Everyone was crying except me. A wave of calm in a sea of turmoil washed over my body. I lay down on the settee and watched the whole scene from somewhere out of myself. Tears couldn't flow because I wasn't there to form them. It was the only way I could cope. I knew there was no point in trying to get to see Steph, as the doctors had already specifically told me that I had to get out of their way if anything went wrong. I couldn't do anything except try to survive myself, which at that moment seemed almost impossible.

The doctor arrived and explained that things had unexpectedly taken a turn for the worse. Stephen had temporarily stopped breathing, which had caused a cardiac arrest. However, the cardiac massage had been successful. He still stood a good chance of recovery, but he couldn't breathe without artificial help. They had stabilised him and were moving him to Intensive Care.

Dad started asking the question that we all wanted to know the answer to. 'For how long was Stephen's brain starved of oxygen? If he recovers . . .' He choked on his own words.

No one wanted to finish the question for him. I thought that they were probably too afraid of scaring me, so I had to come back down to earth and ask the question myself.

'If he recovers, will he be brain damaged?'

As ever, no one could really give me an answer, but he only stopped breathing for seconds. Apparently, he stood every chance of being all right.

We had to wait for Stephen to be settled in Intensive Care before we could see him again, and we were warned that it would take a while to get him hooked up to all the monitors. I decided that it was time for us to start praying out loud. Not that we hadn't all been praying before, each in our own individual way, but at that particular moment in time we were all stuck in the little room together and there was nothing more useful we could do. I had gone to church off and on for much of my life, but had never particularly discussed my faith with anyone. Normally I would have felt embarrassed at suddenly demonstrating a belief in prayer in such a dramatic way, but at that moment I didn't care. Anything was worth a try.

Even the doctor who had been in charge of Stephen began to focus his mind on other things. Steph's care was now out of his hands, so he turned his mind to us. He wanted to know if we'd been given drugs to protect us from contracting meningitis ourselves. My father and I confirmed that we'd each been given a course of three tablets, but that no one else had. Again, the doctor checked that I wasn't on the pill. He was anxious that what I had been prescribed would reduce its effectiveness. For the third time in two days I found myself explaining to a total stranger that we were trying for a family. I told him that I thought I might be pregnant. He looked most concerned and suggested that perhaps I should have been given an injection instead of the tablets, but, as I'd started taking them, I should finish the full course. I was worried, but thought I'd better do as the doctor ordered. I supposed any damage was already done.

After what seemed like an age, we were told to make our way to the Intensive Care ward on the top floor. I tried to get up but my stupid legs wouldn't work, so they had to fetch me a wheelchair. I was annoyed enough at my body for packing up, I couldn't afford for my brain to go too. Stephen needed me more than ever. He couldn't do anything for himself. I had to do it all. Well, almost. He was there inside my head, his voice mercilessly pounding away, *You said you'd survive. You said you'd cope. You said you'd carry on. Just think, Diane, think. Think of all the conversations we had. It's not as though you weren't prepared. I believe you can do it, even if you don't. That's why I married you, remember. You have to keep going.*

In my heart I believed that I was losing him, but at the same time my head told me that I usually worried needlessly. It has since been explained to me by doctors who should know about these things, that when we are afraid of something the human mind projects us into precisely that situation. It is our body's way of facing it, preparing us and teaching us how to cope in the event of it ever happening. At the time I didn't know the psychological explanation, but I realised that my fears were probably an overreaction.

I would have done anything just to be able to press a button, stop the world and take a couple of days off. By then Steph could have turned the corner and be on the road to recovery. On the other hand, what if the worst should happen?

Steph and I had discussed that scenario, and we had agreed about what we would want to happen. It now seemed such a remarkable coincidence that only a few months earlier a newspaper article had been printed about a widow who wanted to have a baby using her deceased husband's sperm. In a way, it was not so remarkable that we had seen it because I was always looking for articles about babies because of my public relations work for Clippasafe nursery products – which my husband often helped me with. We had discussed the article in detail, imagining how we would feel if we found ourselves in that situation. Steph said he hoped that I would still have the opportunity to have his child, even if he were no longer here, and I confirmed that I would be willing, indeed happy, to do that. What I didn't imagine was the effect that conversation would have on the rest of my life. If it hadn't been for that article, I would never have thought to ask the doctors if it was possible to take some of Steph's sperm and freeze it for later use.

But at that moment, I knew it was now or never. I was really scared that the doctors would think I was completely barmy, and I couldn't face any more emotional battles, but I had to ask – for Steph. It's what we'd agreed.

CHAPTER 4

Losing the love of my life

The first person I told was my dad. I wanted him to tell the doctor that I had something to ask and to get us into a position where we could speak privately. Considering I was still incapable of walking, this was about all I could manage. At first my dad seemed a bit shocked, probably because he was given no opportunity to think it all through. I think he was still reeling from the news of Stephen's cardiac arrest and he was amazed that my mind could go off at such a tangent. It didn't seem that way to me because Steph and I had discussed it before. I was just carrying out what we had previously agreed upon and I didn't need time to think. I knew how we had felt at a time when things were far more relaxed and when I was likely to have been in a far more rational state of mind than I was at that particular moment. I just about coped with living through the unimaginable precisely because I had tried to imagine my husband's death when he had been there with me and when we could make all sorts of decisions together about that difficult time. This included the option of maintaining the opportunity to still have a child together.

My father was looking at things from a different perspective. He'd had no time to think or consider what I was suggesting at all. Still, he tried to be open-minded and adjust. He set up the discussion and both he and the doctor listened intently. They didn't appear to think I was nuts, although the doctor had never heard of extracting sperm from someone in a coma. He was concerned that the article I was referring to must have been fiction, but I assured him that it was reported in a newspaper or magazine and purported to be truth. He wanted to know when I had seen it, perhaps thinking it might be a very new procedure. I gave him an approximate date of late summer, early autumn the previous year and all the details I could remember. I told him that I didn't expect him to know all the answers, but that I wanted him to go away and find out. I wasn't going to be fobbed off just because no one had asked the right specialists. It was late evening and there probably wasn't a lot he could do until morning, but the doctor seemed sincere when he promised to go away and find out. I thanked him.

When I first visited Steph on the IC ward, my heart was breaking. He looked OK and the tubes and machines didn't particularly distress me. In fact, I felt much better now he was stable. Now I could relax slightly, I had more tender concerns. Up to this point, the urgency of dealing with Steph's illness had stripped away any chance of intimacy, so I hadn't realised how much I was missing being close to him. Due to the barrier nursing, I was not allowed to touch my husband's skin or hold his hand without the protection of surgical gloves. I had been left in the desert for two whole days and one long night. Anyone who has ever loved someone dearly will understand the craving. It is like an all-consuming thirst that takes hold of the whole of your being. I was craving the touch of my husband's skin. If only I could have stroked his arm.

It was going to be another long night. Sue, one of Stephen's sisters, and her husband arrived, and we were allocated two bedrooms on the IC ward. I took one bedroom and Steph's mum took the other. I so desperately wanted to escape for a while. I pleaded with the doctors for some sleeping tablets, but they couldn't prescribe them for me without consulting my GP. I thought it was ridiculous that I was in a hospital, desperately in need of help, and there was nothing anyone could do.

I shut myself in the bedroom and prayed. I prayed really hard. First, I prayed that my husband would get better, but I also prayed that it would be possible to take a semen sample and that it wouldn't be affected by his illness. If Steph did recover, the frozen sperm might still be useful. I didn't know how and if his future fertility might be affected by either the disease or its treatment. I would have prayed that I was already pregnant, rendering the sperm less important, but for the crippling pain in my stomach. I knew that it was not a good omen. My brain was going into overload and I wasn't sure which would explode first – my head or my stomach.

A few hours into the night, my dad knocked on the door. He'd managed to get me a sleeping tablet. I took it. It didn't knock me out, but I did rest for the brief time I slept. By the morning I felt refreshed enough to just about cope with the devastation caused by the arrival of an extremely heavy period. More bad news was to follow.

The doctors said that my husband's condition hadn't improved during the night. Some of his other organs had started to fail and they had withdrawn sedation to try to get him to breathe on his own. Sadly, he hadn't been able to. He was still relying on the ventilator. Everyone still hoped he would recover, but it wasn't looking good.

I requested a meeting with the doctors in private and we moved to another room. Again I asked about the possibility of taking the semen sample. I didn't want them to think I'd changed my mind and I wanted to know if any progress had been made. To my surprise, they already had some answers. Not only had they discovered that it was possible, but a foremost expert in the field just happened to be in the hospital at the time. I didn't want to get my hopes up. I knew there were no guarantees anyway, but the last thing I wanted was to manage to get the sperm only to be told later that I couldn't use it because it would endanger the health of either myself or our child. I asked if there was any way that the sperm could be affected by meningitis. It could not. What about anything else? The drugs he'd been given? Any other problems relating to his illness? They'd check. They'd do some more tests, but it would take time. I wanted to know before the sperm was taken, but I was concerned that if he died in the meantime, the life-support machine would be turned off. They said that it wouldn't be turned off unless the machine was needed for someone else, which seemed fair enough. Anyway, he wasn't dead yet.

It possibly sounds as though I was giving up on Steph more easily than the doctors. I wasn't. I was just preparing for the worst. I had had all night to think things through and I was focusing very hard on getting it right, both for myself and for Steph. If he died, I knew there'd be no second chances and I had to cover everything.

Now knowing that it was possible to take the sperm, it was time to consult my mother and Stephen's parents, who had begun to wonder what the huddled meetings were about. They were a bit surprised, but they were all in agreement about taking the sperm. I left it up to Stephen's mum to explain the situation to his two sisters, Sue and Bev. Bev, his younger sister, had just flown in from Germany and had arrived at the hospital that morning. Apparently they had already guessed what was going on. Perhaps they had overheard something or they had read similar articles to the one Steph and I had discussed. They certainly knew of their brother's affection for children and the importance he placed on having them.

'We know, it's OK,' one of them said as the other gripped hold of my arm tightly and forced a reassuring smile.

I then went to tell Steph. Apparently, when someone is dying, the hearing is usually the last thing to go. So I told him that we were going to take some of his sperm and that I would still try to have his baby even if he died. It was a precious time, like the calm at the epicentre of a storm. A female doctor sat in the room monitoring him constantly. The machines blipped rhythmically and the ventilator eased breath in and out, making Steph's chest rise and fall in time with the sound. My heart still needed quenching. I longed so much just to touch his skin. I was choked, but I couldn't cry. I remember asking the doctor if she knew the reason for this. I thought that working on Intensive Care she must have talked to lots of relatives in my position. Of course, everyone is different, so she had no explanation. Most people cry. I wasn't numb. It was just that the pain was too sharp, a bit like being cut with a razor blade. It takes a while for the blood to flow. Or when you open your mouth to scream, but the sound doesn't form.

Back in the little suite of relatives' bedrooms and waiting room, my mother had found the tea-making facilities and was doing her best to look after everyone. Meanwhile, I was taken aside and counselled on the details of sperm extraction and infertility treatment. I was told that if I was successful and a child was born, I wouldn't be able to name my husband as the father on the birth certificate. This seemed a bit daft to me, but it didn't seem that important at the time. I had far more urgent things to worry about.

I was told about the success rates and about new forms of treatment. Even if we could only get one sperm and it was of such poor quality that it wasn't even moving, they would be able to inject it into an egg and possibly achieve fertilisation. If they couldn't extract my husband's sperm by the planned method of electro-ejaculation, then even that wasn't the end of the road. They could take testicular tissue and maybe 'grow' the sperm from that. But, at the end of the day, the success rates, if we managed to get the sperm, were still only in the region of between 13 and 25 per cent, depending on the type of treatment. I was asked how I would feel if it didn't work. I was actually surprised the success rates could be so good and really hoped the sperm extraction would be successful. I was then told they'd be bringing across some forms for me to sign from the local fertility hospital to indicate my consent to the procedure. I was quite happy with all the arrangements.

The counselling was informative, but tedious, because it kept me away from my husband when I wanted to be at his side. I tried to listen intently because I knew Steph would have wanted me to. If it meant sacrificing our last hours together then I knew he would understand, so long as I was carrying out the wishes he had previously expressed to me. The future was important, not just the present. I still hadn't been told that he was going to die, but somehow, within myself, I sensed that he wasn't going to make it.

Eventually it was all down to waiting for the results of the tests. I'm surprised my husband had any blood left in his body. They'd already tested it for everything under the sun. I was frightened to death that it would show some other problem that no one had expected, but neither I nor the doctors wanted to take the sperm until we were absolutely sure it would be OK.

It was a long, long wait. I prayed and prayed and prayed. Eventually the news arrived, around 20 hours after I'd first asked about taking the sperm. I was already sitting alone in one of the bedrooms so the doctor didn't need to ask to see me privately. He just knocked at the door and entered with a big smile on his face. 'Everything's fine. You've got the all-clear.'

I was surprised to find that I could cry after all – with relief.

I immediately went to give Steph the good news. I sat holding his hand through the protection of the surgical gloves. 'You can't go just yet, baby. There's one last thing you've got to do. Give it your best shot, please.'

The female doctor obviously overheard. It was a fairly small room. She couldn't really avoid it. 'Actually, we now think there may be a problem,' she interjected.

'What? There can't be a problem, not now.' I'd only just been told it was OK. 'What sort of a problem?'

'Well, we don't know, but it now looks like we won't be able to go ahead.'

I felt as though I'd been punched in the stomach. I'd held my breath for 20 hours, whilst waiting for the results of all the investigations. We'd been given the go-ahead. I hadn't even had time to breathe out. Now this. The blow was crippling. It was totally unbelievable. I'd carefully discussed everything with my family, missed spending time with my husband whilst I was given counselling and, most importantly of all, I'd kept Stephen updated with every bit of good news as it happened. Now the doctor casually slipped out this devastating piece of information, in front of my husband, as though she were telling me that unfortunately she might not be able to meet my invitation to Sunday lunch.

My first thought was whether or not Stephen had heard what she had said. I didn't know if he could still hear. I tried not to get too upset whilst in the room for his sake. I wanted to tell him not to worry. I'd sort it out. But what if I couldn't sort it out? I would need to tell him the plans had been changed. What if he could hear? What if he couldn't? It was doing my head in. I needed to get out.

I turned to make my escape, but my exit was blocked by a group of men. They confirmed that there might be problems and they now weren't going to take the sperm after all. They didn't know what sort of problems. These were a new set of people that I hadn't seen before. I couldn't believe what was happening. It was no time, or place, to be looking into 'possible' problems. I'd just been through all that with the other people who'd counselled me. Did they know we'd discussed things like my husband not being able to be named on the birth certificate? Did they know I still wanted his child anyway?

I said that I wanted legal advice, but I pleaded that it was stupid to be going through this now. They'd had 20 hours to look into all that and they'd told me it was fine. Now we were just wasting time. My husband was dying and we couldn't keep waiting. It seemed to me to make sense to take the sperm now and sort out the problems later. As no one could tell me what they were, I imagined they must be general concerns which could be overcome, rather than any one thing in particular.

I saw a gap between the bodies and went for it. I flew out of the hospital ward and back into the relatives' waiting room, blurting out to my mum what had just happened. She sent someone else in to calm me down while she went to look for my father, who had gone for a walk outside.

He came back in and charged into Stephen's room, tackling the doctor and accusing her of being unprofessional. He was just about to start on the others when the man with the expertise to take the sample stopped him in his tracks by saying that it didn't matter about potential problems, they'd decided to take the sperm anyway. Knowing when to shut up, my father promptly left to relay the good news to me. It was like someone turning off the tap when you're just about to drown.

I had to go back into the room, so the doctors could tell me for themselves. I asked if they had the forms for me to sign, but apparently they hadn't arrived. I don't think anyone fancied any further delays, so the female doctor led the chorus by asking the question, 'We don't care about forms, do we?'

We all agreed that we didn't and my verbal consent was given, witnessed and recorded in the hospital notes. I assumed that the consent I gave was valid and the only one necessary to be given. No one mentioned anything about Stephen's consent and I assumed that, as his next of kin, I was qualified to give consent on his behalf.

I had a few more words with Steph, asking him to do his best, before leaving the room for the doctors to perform the electro-ejaculation. They didn't tell me much about the procedure, except that it was the method of semen extraction commonly used with paraplegics. It couldn't harm Steph and he wouldn't feel anything, as he was in a coma.

It seemed to take no time at all before they were out to report how it had gone. Unfortunately it was very bad news. They had only managed to get a very small sample and it had gone back into the bladder, which sometimes happens with this particular process. They had retrieved the sperm, but they warned me that, although it was not uncommon for them to have to retrieve sperm from the bladder, usually in these cases it was discovered that the urine had killed the sperm and rendered it useless. I did wonder how my husband could possibly have had any urine in his bladder, as he'd had a catheter fitted, but I didn't raise the point. I was more concerned about finding out when and if we could have a second attempt.

More bad news. My expert in the art of sperm removal was just about to leave to go and deliver a lecture in Bournemouth. What's more, he was already late and he wouldn't be back until Saturday. It was only Wednesday night. Putting my embarrassment aside, I grovelled and pleaded every which way I knew how to get him to return sooner and try again, but he was resolute. The only glimmer of hope was that he'd asked a colleague to watch the procedure to try and teach him how to perform the task in the future. Maybe he could have a go. If the attempt failed and my husband was still on life support, then there was always Saturday.

I didn't hold out a great deal of hope of Stephen lasting till Saturday. It seemed his spirit – his sparkle, his energy – had already departed. Machines were carrying out his every bodily function. I accepted that I was going to lose him. I was devastated, but at the same time somehow relieved that his fight and all his suffering was over. I was just so tired. I couldn't imagine us holding out till Saturday. I thought there was more chance of the doctors being totally wrong about the sperm, it suddenly multiplying in quantity and being perfectly fine after all! Accordingly, that's what I prayed for.

Later that same evening the doctors performed the first of two tests to see if Stephen was clinically dead. It was not good news and the emotional exhaustion was by now also beginning to get to Stephen's family. Again, I asked the doctor in charge of Intensive Care about the chances of keeping Steph on life support, explaining the significance of Saturday. So long as the machine wasn't needed for anyone else they would leave it switched on, although, in any event, it could not be turned off before the second test had shown my husband to be dead and the two tests had to be a minimum number of hours apart.

Stephen's parents were devastated and about all-in. They indicated their acceptance that he had passed away and we began to focus on the practicalities of who should be informed and the kind of arrangements that needed to be made for the funeral.

I was lucky because, like most things to do with death, Steph and I had discussed our funeral arrangements in what some might see as a macabre amount of detail for such a young married couple. I was horrified by the thought of being cremated myself and, if I wasn't the first to go, I wanted Steph to have a proper grave that I could go and visit. Steph, on the other hand, had a terrible fear of suffocation and being buried alive. This did not make for a natural compromise on the subject of burial or cremation. However, we definitely both wanted to be laid to rest together, so we'd decided on burial with the caveat that Steph wanted to be buried with a shotgun, in case he woke up. The only problem was that I didn't have a shotgun and Stephen's parents naturally didn't feel very comfortable with the thought of me putting loaded firearms in his coffin.

Instead, I went to ask the doctors if they could confirm without any doubt that he was dead. If they hadn't doubted my sanity before, they certainly would now, but it was something else I had to ask because it was important to Steph. Not that I really needed to ask. You know in your heart the moment when a loved one departs and, looking back, I think I always knew Stephen was going to die. I had known from the moment we sat on the edge of our bed together at home, as we prepared Steph to go in the ambulance. What passed between us in that moment was very profound. It was like an unburdening of the spirit: something Steph gave to me which spoke far louder than words. Its voice cried out through the void, charging me to take good care of our dreams and to carry on as we had planned and discussed. I could hardly go to pieces when I'd promised I'd be OK. That one thought gave me enormous strength.

It seemed logical to have the funeral in the church where we'd married. Actually, Steph and I had never discussed that detail, but the idea met with universal approval. The only problem would be when it came to hymns. It wasn't the most avant garde of churches. They'd been a bit shocked at our wedding when we'd chosen 'Lord of the Dance' as one of the hymns (in the days before Michael Flatley and his Irish dancers had made it famous). We'd also dispensed with 'Here Comes the Bride' and the traditional Wedding March for after the ceremony, swapping them for a couple of more unusual classical pieces.

For his funeral, though, Steph's request was not very classical at all. Led Zeppelin's 'Stairway to Heaven' was the specified song. I had particular problems explaining this in the hospital because, whilst everybody knew that Led Zeppelin were a heavy rock band, no one could recollect that particular song, and my efforts at singing it didn't seem to jog any memories. I think they all had visions of head-banging in the aisles and they tried to be subtle about trying to persuade me that this was not a good idea. I was surprised no one could remember 'Stairway to Heaven'. It was 'our song' – a bit like our version of the last waltz. It had always been the last song played on a Friday night at the heavy metal disco run by one of Stephen's friends that we used to frequent virtually every week when we were courting. It wasn't as though it hadn't been played enough in our respective homes. We both had copies of the record before we were married. In the end, we had to put the subject aside until we returned home and everyone could hear the song for themselves.

Stephen's parents decided to go home the following day. They were worn out and saw little point in hanging around just waiting for a machine to be turned off. They went to say their last goodbyes to their son. I could understand them wanting to go. I did too. The emotional strain was taking a severe toll. There was almost a sense of relief that we could all rest at last.

Finally remembering about my personal hygiene, I decided to go and take a shower in the bathroom provided in the relatives' suite. I felt somewhat refreshed. If only it were so easy to wash away the past four days.

Steph's sisters and I then decided to venture outside for a walk. It had obviously been snowing over the past few days and the world was whitewashed. It was quite a shock because, in the closed environment of the hospital, I'd had no idea what was going on outside. We walked for quite a distance up to some offices where I used to work a long time ago. It was strange. Steph had taken me there the weekend before my interview for the job. We'd gone up to recce the place and walked up to the local shops to get a feel for the area. Now I was walking around those same streets again and he was no longer here.

The day seemed to pass more quickly than the others. Perhaps because we were no longer on tenterhooks. Other relatives came and went, most taking their turn at Steph's bedside to say goodbye; others deciding that they didn't want to see him hooked up to all the machinery. Finally, the doctors arrived again. They were very matter-of-fact. The news was not about Steph but about the sperm samples.

'We're just going to take another sample, but when the last one was processed it turned out to be fine after all. In fact, it was a million times better than we expected, so this is just the icing on the cake.'

So that was it. It seemed my prayers about the sample had been answered after all. There was no great drama. They took the second sample and also did the second test for clinical death. He was dead and the sperm was alive. No one got upset or excited. It was just kind of peaceful.

The doctors then asked for my permission to turn off the life-support machine. I was enormously grateful that I'd never had to make the decision of whether to leave the machine turned on just to retrieve the sperm. Ethically, it's not something either I or Stephen would have had a problem with, as long as it didn't prevent another patient from using a machine they might have needed, but we were all so tired. Emotionally, I don't know if I could have coped with any more.

I was asked whether I wanted to go and see Stephen again first, if I wanted to be there as the machines were turned off and if I wanted to see him afterwards. So many decisions.

I decided that I just wanted to go and see him one more time whilst he was still warm and breathing. They could turn off the machines after I left. I did not want to see the mechanical process of death. I had watched its reality over the past few days. I did not need to witness anything more. It didn't seem important.

I can't really remember my final words to Steph. This time I knew he wasn't there, so I didn't need words. I could speak to him with my heart. I would probably have told him about the sperm, but I felt he knew anyway. Somehow I don't feel he'd have left us if it wasn't going to be OK.

The female doctor was still in the room with us. Stephen was looking a bit unkempt. She asked me if I wanted them to give him a shave. On a good day, if my dark-haired husband had a shave in the morning, he had a five o'clock shadow by lunchtime. He now had five days' worth of growth, but he never really liked the process of shaving at the best of times, so I said to leave him be. Again, to be honest, it didn't really seem important.

It was just a body, but it still looked like my husband and the physical pull was still undeniable. I could no longer bear not being able to touch his skin, so in a broken voice I tried to explain to the doctor, telling her that I wanted to remove my surgical gloves. She pulled off her own gloves and mask, declared that she thought all the bugs would have gone by now and then left us in the room alone together.

Before I finally left the room, I removed my husband's wedding ring and placed it on my own finger, 'Don't worry, love, I'll take good care of it.'

CHAPTER 5

Losing even more

The next few days heralded a stream of visitors wishing to pass on their condolences. Half of them, including my most persistent unwanted Valentine card-sender from my school days, were already at my parents' house when we arrived back from the hospital.

I was grateful for their cards and sympathy, but I was amazed at some of the comments I received. I think people must try extremely hard to search for something positive out of a situation which they really know is anything but. You would be surprised how many told me how lucky I was not to have any children. They said that I shouldn't worry because I would meet someone else. I found this totally bizarre. Didn't they realise I lived with my husband because I loved him, not because I had some desperate fear of being without a partner?

Others suggested that I should go on a cruise or give up my job and become a travel representative. I thought these people should have known me better. I'd always liked my job, so why should I suddenly want to pack it in? Furthermore, I suffer terribly with both home sickness and travel sickness. I don't like to go away for longer than a week at a time and I'm one of very few people I know who gets ill on an aeroplane, let alone an ocean-going vessel of any kind.

Maybe they were stating what they would wish to do if they were ever unfortunate enough to find themselves in my position. I don't think people should judge what is best for someone else on the basis of what may be best for themselves. I do not believe anyone meant to cause me distress by this, but it was upsetting to think that I was obviously so badly misunderstood. It only served to emphasise that the one person who understood me completely was no longer here.

That first night without my husband, I stayed at my parents', but I couldn't sleep and I wanted to go home. Being in the wrong bedroom just reinforced the trauma I was going through. My parents didn't think it was a good idea for me to go home, but I was going whether they liked it or not, so my mother decided to come and stay with me at my little bungalow for a while.

Going home for the first time was not a particularly pleasant experience. I was upset because I discovered the fence had blown down and Stephen wasn't there to resurrect it. The rooms felt cold and rather uninviting. The Valentine card I'd sent to my husband was still displayed on the units in the lounge. I took it down and put it away. The gift card from the flowers he had sent to me I placed in my purse.

It seemed like I could cope with most things. I watched our wedding video fairly shortly after Stephen's death. I was really eager to see if I had a recording of his voice and the video was the only possibility. I could quite happily look through our photo albums. I didn't even mind tackling Stephen's clothes and sorting many of them out, only the weekend after he died.

What I did have a massive problem with was my clothes. Stephen had bought many of them for me and, as I was lucky enough to be the same size at 28 as I had been when I'd first met him at 16, I still had some clothes which held memories going back an awfully long way. My other major problem was food. I couldn't bear to look in the freezer or go to the supermarket. It wasn't that I wasn't hungry, it's just that when you shop and cook for a couple, you choose those items which you know your partner really likes. Having to make those decisions without considering Stephen really got to me. Not very practical really. I was giving away the contents of his wardrobe, which I didn't really have a problem with, whilst my own wardrobe was full of perfectly good clothes I couldn't bear to look at, let alone wear. Even more ridiculous, if it wasn't for my mother, I'd have starved just because I didn't want to decide what to eat.

They say that if you can just grit your teeth and do something for the first time, you get over it and it becomes easier each time. In my experience, the pain becomes duller, not because it goes away, but because you become used to living with it. I made my first trip back to Sheffield only the morning after Stephen died. I had to go to the Hallamshire to fetch the death certificate. I thought it might remind me of my last journey to Sheffield in the ambulance. My parents went with me, but the trip didn't bother me unduly. On arrival, you have to give the name of your relative, and then sit and wait your turn to be called in for someone to explain the stated cause of death (in Stephen's case, bacterial meningitis) and hand over the certificate. I also had to decide whether I wanted them to do a post mortem. They explained that it wasn't necessary because they were certain of the cause of death but that it might possibly help with research – it was my decision. I said that I didn't mind if they wanted to do any posthumous brain scans or anything like that, but I didn't think that research was a justifiable cause for allowing them to cut his body open. Consequently, there was no post mortem, which I am very relieved about, as years later I discovered that it was routine at that time with any disease affecting the brain to remove it for retention at the hospital. I could unwittingly have buried my husband without his brain. This was another of those moments which was to later come back and haunt me. I find it totally bizarre that, as a wife, I could give my permission for my husband's body to be dissected in the name of research, but that I should have no authority to take his reproductive material for my own use, in accordance with his wishes.

The week before the funeral was taken up with the preparations and with me trying to find a freelance person to do my job at work. Before Stephen fell ill, we'd just presented a creative pitch to East Midlands Electricity against an agency in Leicester and a big Manchester agency. Strangely enough, one of my concepts had featured an image of a life-support monitor on the front. While sitting there at the hospital, I'd wondered if we'd win. It was quite an important account for us and I knew it would make Steph very proud. I learnt we'd won the pitch shortly after arriving home following Stephen's death. Unfortunately, advertising deadlines don't get postponed just because you're not up to doing the job, and my colleague, Tim, was quietly getting buried under the piles of work. I rang a couple of people I used to work with to ask if they could recommend anyone to do my job temporarily and I managed to get some guy up from London who'd just finished a contract. I interviewed him and he seemed pretty good, so we did a deal. Four weeks' work for £3,000. I didn't exactly have any option, but Steph would have gone spare. On a good month, I wouldn't normally earn half that amount.

My only job for the next week was writing and typesetting the order of service for Stephen's funeral. I'd already had a run-in with the lady who came to make the arrangements. She kept suggesting that I leave things to her. They'd do something nice. I didn't want to leave anything to anyone. I wanted to specify the colour of his coffin and I certainly wasn't going to put up with the appalling, sombre design of most funeral service sheets. I wanted one which Steph would have liked. My order of service (when I eventually managed to complete this simple but incredibly difficult task) had a picture of a poppy on the front. It was Stephen's favourite flower. Instead of death, the headline referred to a celebration of life. This, I felt, was much more in keeping with Stephen's view of things.

I thought the details were important. He'd obviously considered his funeral and I really hoped he'd get his wish for a church full of people saying what a great guy he was. As for the Led Zeppelin song, it's really quite melodic for a rock song, so when they'd listened to it, no one had found it as raucous as they'd expected. Just in case it offended anyone, I did get it remixed slightly at a recording studio I knew, to get rid of the slightly more raunchy elements in the last verse. At the beginning, I also mixed in the first half of 'Stay' by Shakespears Sister. This was another song that Stephen had liked enormously and, to be honest, as he lay dying at the hospital, I couldn't get it out of my head. It was sort of my last message to him.

The funeral was the following Thursday. I have never seen so many flowers and the church was overflowing with people. Even the side aisles were packed and the pews were crammed with a sea of faces. You couldn't have got more people in if you'd tried. I was enormously grateful that so many had turned out. One of Stephen's wishes had come true. He had his church full of friends. I just hoped that one day he'd also be granted his desire for me to bear our child.

For that, I had to wait. I was told I could contact the fertility clinic after three months. They wanted me to have a chance to get over the immediate grief before they discussed my plans. I was impatient, not particularly to get on with treatment but just to go and talk about it. I was sure they'd all want to have a go at talking me out of it, so I thought the sooner we could get started on the whole tedious process, so much the better.

I waited my three months out. Each day seemed like a lifetime. My eyes constantly ached, both from tiredness (I didn't sleep terribly well) and from crying. I went back to work after the first four weeks. I couldn't afford any more expensive freelance help and my own claim for my month's sick leave was later dismissed by the Inland Revenue as I was a company director. It was hard to concentrate on writing and designing, but it was good to interact with other people.

On our wedding anniversary I took the day off. I wanted to go to the cemetery but I was upset that Steph's grave was still unmarked. I planned a rather elaborate memorial and hadn't managed to organise it by May. For now I decided to make him a little wooden cross. I was never much good at DIY, but Steph had always enjoyed that sort of thing so he had loads of tools and equipment. I spent the day in our garage sawing a couple of planks of wood and fixing them together with a nail. Steph would have been so much better at making it than me. Finally I took the tooling iron he had bought me for my birthday one year. My heart was breaking as I seared in his name, followed by I ♡ U. My tears burnt my cheeks. They felt so hot that I was sure they too would scald the wood as they fell on it. I missed Steph so much.

My doctor recommended that I meet with a bereavement counsellor. I saw him once, but wasn't enthused by the idea of a repeat visit. I got the feeling that he had a few emotional problems himself. He was keen that I felt I could rely on his support but I knew that I needed to support myself. Perhaps I felt stronger than he had assumed. He said that I seemed to be coping well, and once I told him that I had returned to work, he was happy to discharge me.

Instead I decided to go back to Sheffield to see a counsellor whom I had first met in the Hallamshire at the time of my husband's death. This time I found it a positive experience. He helped me to explore my own emotions, instead of suggesting that there were any answers. I went back to see him many times. I wanted to know when I would feel better. I thought he must know, as he'd counselled many young people who had been bereaved or were living with a terminal illness. I thought that if I had a target date, I could concentrate on getting there. He insisted that everyone is different. Initially we only discussed the loss of my husband, but eventually we also talked about my continuing desire to have his child and the problems I encountered along the way.

For now, my concerns about the problems they might hit me with were relatively minor. I thought they'd probably want to tell me their opinion of society's view of these things. I even wondered if the law might suggest it was a bad idea. I never imagined that it might be forbidden, because I'd already read of it happening.

I spent my weekends at various city libraries. I sent for and studied reports: Hansard Debates, the Warnock Report, the White Paper, the relevant law (the Human Fertilisation and Embryology Act 1990), the Human Fertilisation and Embryology Authority's (HFEA) Code of Practice and every infertility medical ethics book I could lay my hands on. Of course, I could only make my own interpretation of their contents. I couldn't ask anyone else because I didn't want to alert people as to what I was considering. I even used my maiden name to send for the reports from the libraries. I'd already read in a newspaper about one widow wanting to use her late husband's sperm. I didn't want to find myself appearing in a newspaper too.

I could see there might be serious reservations about the kind of treatment I wanted, but could find nothing which expressly prohibited my use of Stephen's sperm. The HFEA's Code of Practice was totally silent on the issue. Along with everything else, I even looked at the issue of consent, but, as I read it, I thought everything would be fine. They were just going to give me a good talking to.

I contacted the clinic after the specified three months, but I didn't get an appointment for almost another two months. Finally, a letter arrived with an appointment date of 25 July. I was elated, but not for long. A couple of days later a further letter arrived (actually dated before the first) which warned of 'problems' we needed to discuss. Oh well, I thought, I suppose this was only what I expected. It's not as though I wasn't armed. By now I knew the ethics books inside out.

I asked my dad to go to the appointment with me because I didn't want to go alone. My parents had already tried to persuade me that raising a child without a husband's help might not be the best idea I'd ever had and we'd already been through most of the arguments you could think of. Of course, I'd spent time with the children of friends and relatives, but that's not the same as having your own. The concern, raised by my parents, which I couldn't really answer, was that I didn't know what hard work it would be looking after my own baby. But then again, neither does anyone else until they have one. I didn't know how hard it would be to watch my husband die, but that didn't mean I'd rather I hadn't married him. No possible objection could sway me. They'd come to the conclusion that I seemed to know my own mind, so they saw it as their duty to support me whatever I had decided. Now I knew I could count on their support. Stephen's parents hadn't commented at all. I don't suppose they thought it was their place to try and influence me, and I didn't think I'd find it particularly helpful to discuss it with them when they were still grieving so much themselves.

It was a bit strange sitting in the waiting room of the fertility clinic. My dad was a bit worried about what the other patients might think of us, as it's not very often you'd see a 28-year-old woman and a 51-year-old man sitting together in an infertility clinic. I didn't really care about their opinions, wrapped up as I was in my own thoughts.

My appointment was with Professor Cooke. He had a kind face and I don't think he relished delivering such cruel words. He told me that he'd asked the HFEA and I couldn't use my husband's sperm because I didn't have his written consent. That was it, no ifs, buts or maybes about it. It was presented as the end of the road. He couldn't treat me and he couldn't hand over the sperm or let me take it abroad. He told me that it was the law. I explained that I'd read the relevant law and, in my view, that wasn't what it stated. I told him that I wanted time to seek my own professional legal advice and I asked for his assurance that the sperm would be preserved in the meantime. He promised that it would and I trusted him. My dad asked about the quality and quantity of the sperm. It made sense to check it was suitable for fertilisation. There was obviously no point in arguing over something that wasn't medically viable. Professor Cooke actually didn't immediately know, but he agreed to test it and write to me with the results.

It was the end of September before I received his letter. Professor Cooke had been out of the country for quite a while after our appointment and he apologised for the delay in getting back to me with the news. I had 47 straws and the morphology was 20 per cent ideal. I wasn't sure what that meant, but I was assured that it was adequate for fertilisation. Frozen sperm is always far from 'ideal'. Under the circumstances and given what I had been told at the time it was taken, the news was good.

The legal battle was on. Now I needed to find a lawyer. Difficult when you daren't tell anybody about what you are trying to do for fear of the news leaking out. But even more difficult when you don't trust anyone to work as hard on the case as you would yourself if only you had the relevant legal expertise. After all, no one could possibly share the same investment in the outcome. After making a couple of very general enquiries, I found myself at a barrister's chambers in Nottingham. He thought he'd found the only answer. The sperm was mine as a piece of property. He advised me to write and ask for it, then I could take it abroad. End of problem.

I wasn't happy with this argument. Before I wrote, I wanted to know if there was a counter-argument. Besides, the sperm was no good to me if they thawed it out first. Everyone seemed to think they just had to find a convenient way around the law and then everyone would bend over backwards to help me. I took the view that it was best to assume the opposite. Besides which, I genuinely didn't agree that property was the only answer. I didn't think we had to 'get round the law' because I couldn't believe the law was that stupid. If this interpretation was correct, I could have treatment with the sperm of a totally anonymous donor, even one who was dead, but not that of my own husband. I was unhappy with the shallow nature of such advice, and I wasn't about to take any action until I'd had time to look into it further.

The pressure was beginning to get to me. Everything took time, and the problems surrounding the use of Stephen's sperm did nothing to improve my concentration at work. I was still finding his death alone difficult enough to cope with. I employed a junior to try and ease the burden and to make me less tied to the office.

It wasn't all horrible. We had great fun working on some lovely campaigns for Hotpoint and East Midlands Electricity. One of our Hotpoint advertisements even managed to win us a 'highly commended' mention in the annual advertising awards, so my creativity obviously hadn't gone totally to pot, but I did find myself increasingly alienated from my friends and employees, purely because I couldn't tell them what was going on. In advertising, the business you create one year generally doesn't pay dividends till the next. We were busy now, but I wasn't going out and getting the work for next year. I was afraid that I would be personally too busy to handle it. I didn't think I'd have time for a job, so I was working on the assumption that we only needed enough work for two. From my employees' perspective, knowing nothing about the battle I was facing, I guess they were wondering which one of them would be getting the push first.

As for my friends, they began to notice that I didn't look too well. They thought I needed cheering up so they tried to drag me out partying. This didn't help because the truth was I was emotionally and physically wrecked. I was working non-stop to try and find a solution to my legal problem. With the exception of my immediate family and the counsellor from Sheffield, I told no one what was going on, as I was so afraid of the story being leaked to the newspapers. It is not that I do not trust my friends, but I thought that they might need to share it with their partners or someone they trusted and so it goes on. Telling the counsellor helped, but it's not the same as being able to explain yourself to the people around you. Close personal contacts need to understand why you are acting in a certain way. If you can't tell them, you have to lie, dodge the truth or avoid them altogether. The latter was by far the easiest option, if not necessarily the healthiest.

My sleep was disturbed too. I was always dreaming. They weren't nightmares. In fact, they always had a successful resolution, but I woke up feeling exhausted because I'd just done the night shift too. Night after night I dreamed about Steph and myself. He was always injured or temporarily mentally impaired, and I had to save him and make decisions for the both of us. Sometimes this included setting aside things that we'd previously considered important. For instance, in one dream we were on holiday. We were lying on a hot beach. Steph was ill and began having breathing problems. I had to carry him off the beach and back up to our chalet where it was cooler and I knew he would be OK. The illness had reduced his weight somewhat, so it was possible to lift him, but I also had the problem of having to carry our possessions. I couldn't manage them and Stephen too. I spent a while trying to figure out how to hold on to them both, but I couldn't. Luckily, there just happened to be a wardrobe on the beach. It had a lock, but no key. I put our stuff in the wardrobe, carried Steph indoors and hoped our belongings would still be there when I returned.

Another night, Steph was left seriously ill and in sole charge of a sinking ship, which I had to find and bring safely to shore. It's strange how my subconscious could come up with so many illustrations of the same point. I knew it was all down to me to fight for the both of us. I didn't need reminding. However, on the scale of 'strange but true', these dreams didn't even begin to score compared to what followed. Strangest of all has to be the morning I woke in the early hours feeling absolutely desolate. I missed the physical contact of my husband. I was going through hell, the bed was big and empty, and I needed someone to comfort me. I sobbed and sobbed and sobbed. I was physically sick because I couldn't breathe and then I went back to bed and sobbed some more. I just wanted someone to hold me. I really thought I was going to choke.

'Please, God, please calm me down. I need to breathe.' I certainly couldn't speak, so the words formed in my head.

'Please, God, help me,' I rasped, trying to draw in oxygen.

'Please, God, please send someone to hold me – anyone. Please make it better. Please hold me now.'

Gradually the tears stopped and I drifted off to sleep. But not for long.

My consciousness was shortly aroused as I tried to stop my body sliding downhill towards the slight indentation that had just been created in the mattress to my right-hand side. I tensed my body to stop it rolling but only for a second, then the mattress evened out. Someone had climbed into bed at my side. They'd sat down, twisted around and I'd felt a slight draught as they eased their legs under the quilt.

I was petrified. I wondered if someone had broken into my bedroom with the intention of stealing my jewellery, realised I had nothing worth taking and decided to rape me instead. I lay absolutely still. I couldn't reach the burglar alarm's panic button at the side of the bed because the intruder was in the way. I thought it best to pretend I was asleep.

Then it struck me. I was too close to the edge of the bed. I was lying on my right-hand side, with five feet of empty mattress behind me. There surely couldn't be room for anyone else between me and the edge of the bed. I inched forward slightly, feeling for the edge, but instead I felt just a warm embrace, as a pair of arms wrapped themselves around me. I ceased being afraid for my safety, but I couldn't work it out. I concluded that I must be dreaming. Perhaps I was dreaming about Steph. But I knew it wasn't Steph. Apart from the fact that he was on the wrong side of the bed, I think I would have sensed his presence, even in a dream.

So who was it? They must be awfully thin. I continued to feel for the edge of the bed. As I edged forward, the embrace became warmer, slowly seeming to pass through my body, increasing in both heat and intensity as it did so. It was like being held from within. I have never experienced a grasp so concentrated and profound. I expected the passage to continue and the embrace to disappear out of the back of my body, but it came to rest when the back of their body was level with the front of mine. I thought about opening my eyes, but I figured that it would only make the sensation disappear and I didn't particularly want that to happen.

The only problem was, I still wasn't sure whether this was a dream or reality and I had to find out. I was sure that as soon as I moved my arms the feeling would go, but I couldn't just lie there. Gradually I lifted my left arm, raising it to touch the back of this person's head. Nothing happened. Their grasp remained as intense as ever. I wanted to feel their hair. It was short and extremely fine, like a baby's hair. I wondered why I could touch this silken hair if I was only dreaming. The sensation was very real. There was only one thing left to do: open my eyes. I decided to leave my hand where it was so that, when I opened my eyes, I would at least know that I hadn't dreamt about moving my arm or touching their hair.

Opening my eyes was fairly difficult. It temporarily felt as though they'd been glued shut, but my perseverance paid off and the lids opened. As they did so, the embrace tingled away into thin air, leaving only emptiness and a certain lightness of being. I caught a glimpse of it vanishing: little stars as though Tinkerbell had waved her magic wand in the children's fairytale. My left hand was resting on my own forehead, not quite in contact with it, but touching the ends of the fine, raised little hairs that were standing up on my skin. It was a very strange experience. Perhaps I shouldn't have prayed for anyone to come and hold me. At church, the vicar was always telling us that we should be careful that we really want what we pray for. Me, I thought I'd better go on holiday and take a break before I finally went completely bananas.

So that's what I did. I had no shortage of people volunteering to go with me, but I wanted to go alone. As a bit of a compromise between solitude and company, I spent a long weekend visiting a friend in Swanage on the south coast, went for a day trip to the Isle of Wight with her and then went on my own to a health farm in Leicestershire for five days. It did me the world of good. I must be the only person in the world who could go to a health farm and manage to put on weight instead of losing it. I only gained a couple of pounds, but everyone said I looked better for it.

My employees perhaps thought so too, because they didn't seem to think it would affect me too much when, only a couple of weeks after I returned, they both handed their notice in within a week of each other. One went to one of my suppliers; the other to a client, taking with him both their future business and £4,185 worth of advance media bookings which I had thought secure as they'd already been negotiated and placed through my company. Once my account executive took up his new position, these were handled directly by the client. Losing business along with staff is one of the dangers of the advertising industry, but it's often a client that the employee has brought in themselves. In this case he'd not even met them or had anything to do with them until my husband died.

I was going to employ another account executive as a replacement, but I couldn't quite bring myself to do it. I was afraid of beginning to work with a stranger when I had so many other complicated things going on in my life.

I went to see a firm of solicitors on the Embankment in London, wondering if posh city offices might make their advice any more comprehensive. Over two days, I poured out my story to a young solicitor named Mark Tudor. I quite liked him. He seemed sympathetic, he had a young family of his own and appeared enthusiastic enough to explore different avenues and not look at my case with tunnel vision. The company was therefore appointed as my solicitors.

On 15 December, the HFEA sent them their new Code of Practice to accompany the Human Fertilisation and Embryology Act 1990. It explicitly addressed my particular situation and stated that fertility treatment was forbidden unless the man had given consent to the posthumous use of his sperm. In those cases, it would be regarded as treatment using the sperm of a donor. Consent was also required for export. This was their new interpretation of the law, not the law itself, but if I didn't challenge the Code within three months it would stand. I had to act quickly or it would be too late to do anything about it later.

Things were pretty hectic and I hadn't improved matters with my earlier decision that I didn't want a run-of-the-mill headstone for Stephen's grave. In life, he had a particular taste for expensive watches. I'd always promised to buy him one some day, but I'd never got round to it. That's why I decided that his headstone would be a sundial. I'd designed it myself, taken an absolute age writing a poem for his epitaph and was currently having difficulty commissioning all the bits to get it finished in time for Christmas.

Work was getting ridiculous. I couldn't handle it all myself and I knew that I was temporarily incapable of making someone else's business my number-one priority. As I've already said, when you run an advertising agency, deadlines have to come before everything else in your life. If you're not there to meet them, you have to know and trust that someone else will. I was no longer in a position to do that, so, rather than let anyone down, I resigned most of my business and farmed some out to an agency I used to work for in Nottingham, giving them all the profit in the hope that I could retain the client when my legal problems were sorted and I had more time.

Resigning business may sound like the coward's way out, but it was a very tough decision to make and even harder to execute. Imagine handing in your notice when you really enjoy your work and get on with the people you work with, then multiply it by however many clients. It's bad enough leaving a job you like when you know you're going to one you'll enjoy more. I was giving up my clients for no job, no salary and, worst of all, I couldn't give them an honest explanation for my actions.

Christmas 1995 was pretty dire. We did get the sundial finished. It was erected on winter solstice in the middle of a snowstorm. This, I think, was my lowest point. I'd shut out all my friends because I couldn't talk to them. I'd lost my business, my husband and I had no faith in any legal argument I'd heard so far. I even began to question my faith in God. I didn't think He'd allow this to happen to me. I went to the little church at the bottom of my road and sat there in the middle of the carols with tears streaming down my face. I was no longer convinced that Jesus existed, but in the hope that He did, I asked for His help.

CHAPTER 6

The faint ray of hope

The new year got off to a reasonable start. I'd been waiting for some independent expert advice from Derek Morgan, co-author of *Blackstone's Guide to the Human Fertilisation and Embryology Act 1990*. It was the only book that had ever really tried to dissect and decipher the Act, so if anyone could understand it, it would be this man. I was supposed to get the advice before Christmas, but it had taken longer than he expected. When it arrived, it was worth the wait. It was the first ray of hope that anyone had proffered. He could see several ways of attacking the HFEA's stance. He supported the view that the sperm could be taken abroad as my property, but there were also other routes which warranted further exploration. He even thought that I might be able to get treatment in England.

A barrister from Inner Temple was also consulted for his opinion on the case and he helped draft a letter to the HFEA, asking for clarification of their opinion. We asked if they would allow treatment, either in this country or abroad, with my husband's sperm. The letter went off.

I was pleased with the progress and I took Derek Morgan's report with me when I went to visit my sister-in-law, Bev, shortly afterwards. She'd just moved back to Berkshire from Germany, but her husband was away and she was finding it a bit hard, as she didn't really know anyone in her new town yet. I thought we could cheer each other up. I told her all about the case. She was concerned that I seemed to be facing such an uphill struggle and was especially alarmed when I told her that, even if I won and had a child, Steph wouldn't be named on the birth certificate. Even so, she understood why I found that relatively unimportant and was pleased that Derek Morgan had offered me a positive view. Naturally, she was still missing her brother deeply. We talked about him a lot and reminisced. It was comforting to share our memories and it was a good weekend, which was just as well, as I needed bolstering up for the next big blow that was about to hit.

A letter arrived from my solicitor, explaining that he was leaving the firm and my case had been passed on to one of the partners. I was absolutely gutted. I felt abandoned. I'd only appointed that firm because I thought he'd been enthusiastic enough to work on the case. I'd spent two days with him reliving the agony of my husband's final hours and now he was passing me on to someone I'd never met. I wondered if he could take my case with him to his new firm but, when I called, I discovered that he'd actually been made redundant, so he didn't immediately have anywhere to go to.

I thought that once I got to know my new solicitor, things would be fine and I'd feel more relaxed, so we made an appointment to go and see him, and my dad and I went down to London to check on the latest progress being made with the case. Dad tried desperately hard to reconcile me to the new guy, but basically we just never really hit it off. He was a senior partner in the firm and their main portfolio was in contract and business law. My case was a very individual personal issue, and if you weighed up the odds on a purely financial basis, you would have had to be deranged to even contemplate taking it to court because it seemed there was no way I could win. It wasn't a claim for compensation and, if we were talking in monitory value, the net value of my husband's sperm was £15. That's the amount a donor would have been paid at the time for donating a sample. If you applied normal logic, my case just didn't add up – unlike the mounting bills. I felt that my new solicitor just didn't appreciate my emotional investment in the outcome, whilst he was concerned about the state of my finances. As a partner, he had kindly offered to work for the same hourly rate as the junior I'd initially agreed on, but then again I'd been quite happy with the less senior solicitor and I hadn't wanted to upgrade. I didn't really know what to do. I couldn't fault the partner's work and changing to an entirely new solicitor was not something I particularly relished the thought of, so the firm continued to represent me.

My barrister, Michael Fordham, I liked and trusted enormously. At our first conference, he'd painfully deliberated over the probability of a successful outcome but finally said that it was difficult to estimate, so I told him not to bother. He later confessed that this was rather a liberating relief, and he was pleased I wanted a barrister rather than a bookmaker. For my part, I wanted him to fight my case, not spend ages worrying about the odds of winning. This was irrelevant to me anyway, as, unless it was absolutely hopeless, I still had to pursue it, otherwise I'd spend the rest of my life never knowing if I could have won.

I also had Lord Lester of Herne Hill QC working on my case from the same chambers. He had done some work on it pro bono, for which I was immensely grateful. Despite their chambers having worked for some pretty famous people, the one thing they couldn't really give advice on was the likely effect of my case hitting the headlines. I was worried that I could win the case, only to find out that treatment would be forbidden because of the effect of possible publicity on the child. The law required the treating clinic to take account of the welfare of the potential child in deciding whether to treat a widow. Also, I didn't know what the public reaction would be. If I was shown universal contempt, then I wouldn't want my child to grow up with everyone knowing the circumstances of their birth. It would have been so much simpler if we could have just banned the news from getting out altogether, but I was also afraid of it being reported with only half the facts. The HFEA would be able to give their version and people would not have the opportunity to hear my reasoning. In the end, we decided that, if we had to go to court, we would ask for an anonymity order to protect just my name and the name of the town where I lived. To be honest, I was told that to get an order covering other details would be extremely hard, if not impossible, in any event. The best bet was just to keep quiet and hope that no one found out.

By the beginning of March 1996, I was beginning to get particularly anxious that the HFEA hadn't responded to our letter. We'd chased them up on it several times, but there was still no response. Time was moving on. There was obviously no point in going through the costly process of issuing a writ if they were going to allow treatment, but under the procedural rules of judicial review (the type of action I was contemplating) I had to challenge the Code of Practice and the basis for the HFEA's decision before the three months were up. The deadline was looming in under a week's time, so my dad and I visited the solicitors again to decide what to do. They thought we should still wait for the response, but I didn't want to run out of time, so I gave instructions to apply for leave to go to court anyway. It's just as well that I did. Without knowing that we already had this prepared, the HFEA finally gave their response on the afternoon before my deadline. It had taken them almost three months to say 'no'.

The papers were submitted to the court immediately and the leave hearing (to decide whether or not the law was in sufficient doubt to even bring a full case to court) was set for 9 May 1996. We asked for it to be considered just on paper without it going to court to save on costs, but the judge wanted a hearing. It was to be held 'in camera', meaning there would be no access for reporters or the general public. I was really concerned that I wouldn't get leave, and I got more and more tense.

The HFEA opposed neither leave nor the anonymity order, but, to add further to the cost, the court appointed a barrister of their own, an amicus curiae, to play devil's advocate and put forward the case for the newspapers being able to freely report everything. The amicus curiae would be paid for by the state, but I still had to pay for my solicitors to copy him with details of the case and to prepare my defence for anonymity when it would have been otherwise unnecessary.

I wondered what Steph would have made of it all. I knew he'd have been worried sick about the potential cost, but I didn't have a choice.

We had to leave quite early in the morning to catch the train down to London for the hearing. I suppose it would have made sense to have a nice early night and go to bed with a cup of cocoa. But I couldn't just sit there doing nothing. Instead, I spent a good proportion of the evening in the Medical Library at the Queen's Medical Hospital in Nottingham, poring over various books and reports trying to see if I could find anything we'd missed. Amongst other things, I searched for opinion polls on IVF treatment for various categories of patient. I was stunned by the lack of professional research into the area and the credibility attached to the various DIY jobs of individual doctors or clinics. Having spent my whole career working in advertising and public relations, I am no particular expert on the field of research, but I do recognise and respect the skill involved in its compilation. I know how easy it is to get a highly inaccurate view just by asking the questions in the wrong way.

The only vaguely relevant piece of research I could find was a Canadian report which was probably too old to be a useful gauge. The report found that the general public of Canada were happier to allow the treatment of single women than the treatment of cohabiting unmarried couples. It was professionally researched, but the book merely reported that this finding was a bizarre anomaly instead of questioning why. Especially given the age of the survey, it seemed to me that those questioned about their opinions might think that a single-parent household was perhaps more stable than one with unmarried parents who had decided not to undertake the full commitment of marriage. I certainly thought that I could provide a stable home for the child I hoped for.

I arrived at the solicitor's the next morning wound up like a spring and armed with at least half a dozen new facts and a new stack of photocopies from the medical books. The solicitor wasn't interested, however, because they weren't legal books. I wanted someone to look at the information I had uncovered before they decided whether it was or was not relevant, but he was concerned about spending, what was in his view, unnecessary time on them. He didn't want to waste my money. I suppose it was fair comment, but it didn't feel that way at the time, as it was my future at stake and a judge was about to give a verdict that could change the course of my life.

We walked across to the barristers' chambers and then across the road to court. The hearing was before the President of the Family Division, Sir Stephen Brown. It was an old-fashioned courtroom, with dark wooden pews and legal books adorning the equally dark shelves that ran the full length of the side walls. It was pretty awesome and intimidating, but the sort of place for which you would have to have respect. We chose a pew and sat down. We imitated the book shelves. My dad propped me up on one side and my mum on the other.

The proceedings got under way quickly. My barrister, Michael Fordham, stood up and asked for leave to go to court. He began to give his arguments, but the judge stopped him mid-sentence to tell him we had leave. He could have given that on the strength of the papers we had submitted, so we were only in court because he was concerned about my request for anonymity.

My sense of relief was overwhelming. The rest was only detail. I had what I wanted. In comparison to being granted leave, the anonymity issue was so insignificant to me that I suddenly wanted to go home and catch up on all the sleep I'd missed.

As I listened to the deliberations, I thought that the judge spoke an awful lot of common sense. Basically, he couldn't understand why I wanted anonymity. He wanted to know what I thought I had to hide. He asked the question several times, but in judicial review neither the applicant nor the defence ever give verbal evidence themselves. It's really frustrating. The judge asks a question as though he's addressing you and your barrister answers for you. I really wanted to scream out and speak for myself. 'Nothing! I've nothing to hide.'

By the time the judge had finished, he'd half convinced me that anonymity was a bad idea. I didn't want people to think I was ashamed and his questions about having nothing to hide rather made me suspect that, by asking for anonymity, I had created that impression. As I've already explained, my biggest fear was that I'd win the court case, only to be told that I then couldn't have treatment because the publicity created by the case would affect the child, but Sir Stephen Brown couldn't understand this one at all. He asked the HFEA for their opinion. They agreed with the judge that they didn't really think the publicity would affect a child and would not affect a decision on treatment.

I have to admit it was like jumping ten steps ahead before we'd got to the first hurdle. The argument for protecting the interest of a child that doesn't exist was, at times, a little tortuous. Sir Stephen Brown also came up with something I'd simply never thought of and no one had suggested to me. If there was a child at some point in the future and publicity became a problem, then I could always go back to that court to request an order to prevent the newspapers from hounding them. He didn't have a problem with giving an order on behalf of a child. He had a problem giving an order to me to protect 'someone' who might not even get the opportunity to be conceived. The judge wanted to solve one problem at a time.

In the end, he gave in to my barrister. I don't really think he'd been convinced of anything. He was quite clear that he would only give an order to protect my name and prevent the publication of my photograph. All other details could be reported freely. To be honest, I think he felt it was no longer worth arguing over something which he didn't believe would achieve a great deal anyway. If everything else was reported, then the person's identity would be of only minor significance. It would be simple enough to deduce who they were from all the other details peculiar to the case. An example of this was the name and address of my GP. We had asked for this to be protected, as it would identify the town where I lived. This was refused.

Our final request – that the case be expedited – was granted. We were given two weeks to submit our evidence and the HFEA four weeks to respond. I was so pleased that, after all the waiting, this was it, something was actually going to happen – quickly. No one could mess me around any longer. They had to respond within a given timeframe, so I wouldn't be left in suspense as I had been when waiting for the HFEA to reply to my solicitor's first letter asking them if I could have treatment.

I went home a very happy lady. The heat was really on to get some answers. Being busy helped divert me from my grief, but it wasn't a method of escape. If it hadn't been the court case that took up my time, it would have been work and the other things I'd had to sacrifice to make way for it. A normal 30-year-old widow wouldn't often have time to wallow in misery and neither did I. The weeks were tolerable. I felt we were getting somewhere and working towards our goal. It was the weekends that really dragged. My parents occupied me by taking me out on lots of day trips. It was better than sitting at home, but I would have preferred to be with Steph. The weekends were obviously when we had spent most time together, so that's when I missed him the most.

We began work on my affidavit and on trying to obtain the evidence I needed. First, we had to find the newspaper article that my husband and I had read and discussed, but it was like looking for a needle in a haystack when you don't even know the location of the haystack. With hindsight, the task shouldn't have been so difficult, but neither my family nor my solicitors knew where to start. I asked around, without giving the specifics, and I discovered that there is a newspaper library near King's Cross. It has a copy of every paper that's ever been printed – a rather large 'haystack'. The problem is that only the broadsheets are categorised and held on CD. If the story I was looking for was printed in a broadsheet, I could search using keywords, but otherwise the only way to find it would be to read every paper. I actually thought it pretty unlikely that it had been a broadsheet, so I tried to find a simpler way before I made the trip.

I went to see Professor Cooke at the Jessop Hospital for Women because I had begun to have slight problems with irregular periods, which he attributed to stress. I asked him about the article while I was there. I was sure that people in the medical profession would be able to remember more particular details of the case that might help pinpoint the article, but, unfortunately, Professor Cooke didn't know of any reported case of posthumous conception.

People respectfully began to suggest that perhaps I was mistaken about the story. It seemed so unlikely that I knew about the case when no one else did. I remained adamant, but I began to think that everyone doubted my word.

Eventually, my solicitor realised that they had a computer system capable of searching for files such as newspaper or legal reports at their offices. Not every newspaper was on it, but it did include some of the tabloids and you could search each publication using keywords. It was very simple. All I had to do was give parameters for the date and a list of possible publications. I actually didn't subscribe to any newspapers myself and didn't have a habitual pattern of buying any. Instead, my husband and I used to read those my parents purchased, which numbered quite a few.

The search was done on these papers and my story was found. I had given the correct approximate date, and the story was carried in the publications my parents subscribed to. There were actually two cases around the same date, and they had been reported in a couple of the newspapers. One was the story of an American lady who had been married only a few months when her husband died in a car accident. Sperm was extracted for her use after his death. The other story was of a British woman who had been impregnated with her husband's sperm following his death from cancer. I had a bit of a problem saying with absolute certainty which particular article had triggered the discussion between my husband and myself. The basic questions they posed were all so similar that any or all could have formed the basis for our conversation, which I remembered with clarity. We had been sitting around our dining table at some point after reading the story. I had said that if I ever found myself in the woman's position, I would still want to have Steph's baby. He said he hoped if such a situation arose that I would be able to have his baby. We decided to submit all the articles in evidence with this explanation. It might have been easier just to pick one and say that was definitely it, but I had to swear an oath on the Bible and it would have been a lie.

My other task in building my case was to obtain several pieces of medical evidence. The English legal system does not operate the way you see in films, when they spend ages deliberating over an interesting but hypothetical theory. If a judgement would not have a practical application, they won't even consider the case, let alone decide the outcome. When you take into account the backlog of cases, and the impact on the learned judges' time, this is really rather more sensible than the Hollywood version of the legal system. All the same, it didn't make for a simple life.

I had to obtain confirmation that a clinic outside the UK would be prepared to treat me, if we could persuade a court, by whatever route, to give a direction that I could take the sperm there. For this, I really needed confirmation from clinics in two countries: one in the USA (where we knew treatment was probably legal because of one of the newspaper reports we'd found) and one in a member state of the European Union. The law might draw a distinction between the two. It would depend on whether we ran with the property argument or perhaps relied on laws which just related to the EU. At the best of times this would be a difficult task; but when you're also trying to avoid the news leaking, it becomes a mammoth undertaking because you have to be so careful who you talk to. I also didn't even know where to start looking for the clinics. In the end, my family and I concentrated on finding a clinic in the USA, and I asked Professor Cooke if he would ask some of his colleagues from clinics in the EU whether they would help me. As Professor Cooke already knew all the details and had done for a long time, he was one of the few people with whom I could discuss the situation.

We discovered that, although the USA has no central legislation on infertility, they do have an appointed authority to oversee the whole area of reproductive medicine. The American Society for

Reproductive Medicine in Birmingham, Alabama, were really helpful. Apart from general advice about their country's law governing fertility treatment, or rather lack of it, they supplied me with a list of all recognised clinics. There were hundreds and hundreds, so I picked a few and wrote to them. My choice was quite random, as none of the names meant anything to me. I chose those on the east side of the USA purely because it was nearer, and picked clinics in different states, in case individual state law had any bearing on their response. Some clinics simply didn't respond, but out of my first batch of letters came two positive replies. The first of these was really refreshing. They genuinely seemed to want to do everything possible to help. It was such a change from the reaction in England, where it seemed that everyone wanted to put up all the obstacles they could find.

Professor Cooke took a little longer to get a response from those clinics he'd approached in Europe, but, finally, Greece came back with a 'yes', subject to us first addressing in Britain the legal ramifications of exporting the sperm and the possible achievement of a pregancy. Obviously, we were doing this. Belgium settled on a definite maybe. They wanted to put it to their ethics committee, but it would take a while for them to consider it carefully and give their answer. We only had two weeks, so we decided to go with Greece. In theory, there was no difference between Belgium and Greece, but we thought it might have sounded better fighting on EC (European Community) law with one of the centres for the EU itself. It was therefore disappointing that they couldn't give a speedier reply.

Possibly the trickiest medical evidence we had to report on was my own suitability for treatment. For this, tests needed to be done at different points in my menstrual cycle. We had two weeks and obviously the menstrual cycle takes four. Luckily, the two weeks fell at the right point in my cycle to fit in a day-21 progesterone test, which proved I was ovulating normally, and some poor unsuspecting Sheffield hospital had to squeeze me in for a tubal patency test on the very day I rang up about it. If they hadn't seen me that day, I would have had to wait another month, by which time it would have been too late. I obviously had to give them some reason for the rush, so I explained it was needed as evidence for a court case, without giving further details.

They were very obliging and managed to fit me in at short notice. The test was to see if my fallopian tubes were open. If they were not, it would have meant I could not have conceived either naturally or with normal artificial insemination. My only hope would have been IVF. Obviously, we wanted my tubes to be open, as this would mean that I stood a better chance of success, with the opportunity to use less invasive methods of reproductive medicine. In order to do the test, they must inject dye into your fallopian tubes and then photograph them. The results of the test can be seen straight away.

The doctor gave me the news, 'Well, I don't know if this is what you want to hear, but both your tubes are fine and open.'

I guess he must have presumed my case was for negligence or injury. I wanted to shout 'Yippee', but I was cautious not to sound too enthusiastic because I didn't want to have to explain what my court case was about. I just told him that he'd given me the result I wanted and left him looking rather bewildered and confused.

All the same, the confirmation that nothing was wrong with my fertility did bring a slight lump to my throat. It meant that, even if I hadn't already been pregnant at the time Steph died, I soon might have been if only he'd lived just a few months longer. There is never a good time to lose a loved one, but it made me reflect once again on the cruel timing of Steph's sudden departure from the world.

At least my evidence finally seemed to be coming together and taking shape. I also found a new firm of solicitors to represent me: Leigh, Day and Co. They were more used to dealing with personal cases and had much more experience of judicial review, the type of action I was taking. After talking things over with my old solicitors, we decided that it would be better if we handed my case over to the company with more relevant expertise. It was an amicable parting and they wished me luck.

The team was ready. My evidence was submitted. We even finally had a date set for the hearing – 2 and 3 October. This was the two days after the summer recess. The courts close during August and September, so I guess the first two days back were the best I could hope for. October seemed a long wait after the rush to submit evidence, but getting the first hearing after a recess does have distinct advantages – at least the case before it can't overrun and delay yours. I was just pleased that it was all arranged and I had something to look forward to. I had a date in my diary and I knew it wouldn't be changed. With that solid piece of knowledge, I thought I could just about hang on in there until then.

CHAPTER 7

Gaining strength for the fight

The summer of 1996 wasn't the best I've ever had. I thought it was going to drag on for ever. The HFEA's evidence, when it was eventually filed towards the end of August, did nothing to elevate my mood. I hadn't really expected it to. I already knew that the HFEA's legal objection was down to my husband's lack of written consent. This prevented storage and treatment in the UK and, although it was within the HFEA's power to permit export, they had issued general directions in 1991 which stated that written consent was also required for export. These general directions also meant that sperm could not be used abroad in cases where it could not be used lawfully in the UK.

What did surprise me was that in a telephone attendance note from 2 March 1995, when Professor Cooke had called the HFEA to discuss my situation, they had recognised that the current situation was 'traumatic' and said 'it would appear uncaring and unnecessarily bureaucratic to insist on proper legal consent at that time'. They advised that 'the man's written consent for storage was a legal requirement and that it needed to be established whether he had given consent in any form at any time'. I now didn't understand why they no longer seemed interested in the fact that it had and I wondered how, having originally given their consent for storage, it could ever be anything other than 'uncaring and unnecessarily bureaucratic' to destoy my husband's sperm later.

I had also not anticipated that ethical concerns would be raised about posthumous conception in general, as it was common ground that this was perfectly legal where there was written consent. I was therefore particularly annoyed that they'd managed to include in their arguments one of those DIY research jobs from a clinic who opposed my point of view. I'd never actually managed to find any research that directly addressed the issue of posthumous use of a deceased man's sperm by their surviving partner, but this one was almost bang on target. It asked for the views of clinics rather than the public, but I couldn't believe the way the questions had been asked. I would have called it a canvass for support of an opinion, not a piece of research at all. Even so, it actually showed that the majority of clinics who replied would support posthumous treatment for a surviving partner. It had been submitted in the HFEA's evidence to demonstrate that a 'substantial minority' would not. I thought I ought to remember that one next time one of my advertising campaigns bombed out on research. 'Well, never mind, Mr Client, I think you should still buy it anyway. A "substantial minority" thought it was really good.'

However, what I found most upsetting about the HFEA's evidence was that I learnt from it that they had held a meeting on 23 May at which they had re-examined the facts of my case and apparently specifically considered whether, in my particular circumstances, it was appropriate to depart from their general directions which forbade export. The decision had not gone in my favour. My evidence had not been submitted until 3 June. How could they have considered the specific facts of our case? They hadn't known what they were and they hadn't asked. Like the HFEA, we had slightly overshot our deadline for evidence, but once we had a date set for the hearing, which was after summer recess in any event, no one had known of any reason to adhere to the original deadlines too strictly. If I'd been aware that the meeting was to take place, I would have welcomed the opportunity to present our arguments. It hadn't occured to me that they would discuss us without consulting either myself or my lawyers first.

Something else which had never occured to me was to seek the backing of a medical expert witness. The HFEA presented evidence from a clinical lecturer in obstetrics and gynaecology at the UCL Medical School, Middlesex Hospital in London. She wasn't strictly independent, as she was actually a paid employee of the HFEA, but at that time we didn't have anyone for my side. We thought we'd better find someone, but this was easier said than done, for two reasons. First, I was still afraid to tell anyone (even doctors) about my case for fear the news would leak and, second, all relevantly qualified infertility doctors are licensed by the HFEA. The HFEA inspect their clinics and have the right to close them down. I could see why opposing them in court might not necessarily be a good career move for the specialist involved. I needed someone who was not afraid to speak their mind, not only in spite of possible repercussions from the HFEA but also in spite of what public reaction may be. This was still an unknown quantity and I did realise that I was asking for rather a lot.

I began to feel somewhat overburdened by what I saw as the unevenness of it all. The HFEA had medical people on tap; I didn't know where to start looking. They were risking their budget; I was risking my home. If they lost, it would affect none of them personally. If I lost, it was an issue of such central importance to my life, that I may as well have been incarcerated. To be denied the freedom to carry out your own will is bad enough; I was also fighting to carry out the wishes of my husband.

For me, everything was on hold. I wanted – no, I needed – the rest of my life back. When something dreadful happens in a person's life, the trail of destruction that it leaves may seem insurmountable. Most manage to work their way through it, and I was managing to work my way through my husband's death. I believe that we are each the author of our own destiny and, therefore, whether or not we cope in the circumstances in which we find ourselves is a personal decision that each person makes. We choose the path we take, and if we get it wrong, then we have no one to blame but ourselves. I think the facility to go your own way and stand on your own two feet is dreadfully important after the loss of a partner. I cannot imagine how widows cope in countries where they are denied that opportunity, being seen only as an extension of their husband. They not only lose the man they love, but also their own identity and voice.

This is how I felt about being denied treatment with my husband's sperm. I couldn't bring him back, but I didn't have to give up on the rest of the plans I had made for my life, or the potential of fulfilling my husband's wishes. If I was ever allowed to have treatment and I failed medically, then that would be a reality that I would have to come to terms with. At least then I would know I had done everything possible. What I couldn't see my way round, through or over the top of, was the enormous hurdle that I currently faced. This was an obstacle created by man, not by nature or by God. I'd entrusted my life to Him, a much higher authority than the HFEA. But, for now, I had to sit tight and wait whilst someone else held all the cards.

Sitting and waiting were not my specialities. With nothing positive to do, I became terribly afraid. I visited my husband's grave regularly and I prayed day and night. When I'd first lost Steph, I could look at other people who'd once been in a similar situation and see that they'd survived, but I had no precedent for my situation with the court case. I really didn't know if I could get through it. The only thing I did know for sure was that if I didn't cope, I would lose everything. There wasn't much point fighting to try and become a single mother if the fight left me drained of the ability to be fit for the job.

I thought it was time for another holiday. It was a year since I'd taken the few days at the health farm and it felt like a lifetime ago. This year I decided to go to Edinburgh for the Festival. I have always adored the theatre. I used to go regularly and had managed to convert Steph to its delights early on in our relationship. Our last trip to the Sheffield Lyceum together had been only a couple of weeks before he'd died.

I sent for the Fringe brochure and scheduled my time with great precision in order to squeeze in as many productions as possible. I had a brilliant time. For once, even the Scottish weather was bright and shiny. Much better than the weather I left behind in England, by all accounts. I had gone alone, but to be lonely would have been impossible. I helped compose and perform an ad-hoc play with a girl from Newcastle and a guy of Indian origin from Edinburgh. I got roped into reading poetry in a pleasant, cobbled little courtyard in front of a poetry library and I watched some really interesting productions.

However, I still managed to leave a few free afternoons and evenings just to sit and watch the world go by. I spent one particularly sunny afternoon just sitting on some steps on the top of the Waverley shopping centre listening to a band give a free performance to try and drum up support for their gig. Another evening I joined a group of teenagers at the bottom of the Royal Mile. They played the guitar and sang rather badly. I sat on the pavement with them, eating my fish and chips, singing 'Wonderwall'.

I recount these moments in time not because they can be recaptured or described with any accuracy, but because I stated at the outset that this book was, in part, a thank you to those who helped to save my life. These people, who I do not know and will never meet again, without knowing it helped me to survive when the pressure was almost unbearable. Their passion for life was infectious.

I once asked a friend what I intended to be a rhetorical question: 'How do you survive, when you think you cannot?' He replied that the alternative was to kill yourself and there were too many books to read, galleries to see, pieces of music to listen to, plays to watch and places to visit to give up on life. These words came from someone who had once attempted suicide and was rather glad he had failed.

I must admit that never in my lowest moment could I have vaguely contemplated physically killing myself, but there were times when I did not think my body could endure such intense pain and anguish. I realised that I was allowing myself to be destroyed mentally, and I couldn't allow that to happen. If I did, then Steph would have no one to fight for him.

I returned from my holiday as psychologically prepared as I could possibly have been for the fight ahead. It seemed that most of my legal team had been on holiday too. When we eventually all returned and reconvened ready to do some work, it was frighteningly close to the hearing date and we still didn't have an independent expert medical witness. We had a conference with the entire team to decide what to do. Richard Stein, my solicitor, had already asked one doctor who we'd been told had once carried out the same procedure as I was looking for prior to the 1990 Act coming into force. It hadn't resulted in a pregnancy and the woman had decided not to continue trying. We had thought he would be sympathetic, but the fertility doctor concerned had since swallowed the HFEA's rhetoric and he thought we might be better looking elsewhere for a witness. He didn't think I would win and seemed to misunderstand what I was looking for. I wanted his professional ethical view, but he appeared to think I was looking for his legal advice. I had my lawyers to provide that. He was not entirely unhelpful. He suggested to my solicitor that we might try Professor

Lord Winston, but with the caveat that he was an incredibly busy man and extremely difficult to get hold of.

So it turned out that three of us turned up at the conference with the same suggestion. My solicitor put forward the view of the doctor he'd already asked. I commented that I thought the professor who featured on the BBC *Making Babies* series that I'd been watching seemed very nice and kind, and my QC, Lord Lester, had read and been impressed with the clarity of argument in an article that Robert Winston had written in one of the papers that morning.

Lord Lester called Lord Winston at the Hammersmith Hospital where he worked. He came to the phone straight away, so we imparted the brief details of the case and asked if he would be prepared to help. He confirmed that he would. I was absolutely delighted. It was so close to the hearing date that I'd almost begun to despair of finding anyone, let alone someone of the calibre of Lord Winston.

We had left Lord Winston with hardly any time to prepare his evidence, so my solicitors organised all the current evidence to be couriered over to him immediately and we arranged a conference with him for the following week. Given Lord Winston's hectic schedule, the fact that he is a devout orthodox Jew and that that weekend was Jewish New Year, it must have taken an amazing feat of time management and dedication to achieve anything at all in the allotted space of time.

When I first met him the following week, I was already seated in the waiting room at the barristers' chambers. My father was with me. Lord Winston arrived shortly after us and took a seat a short distance away from me. Of course, I recognised him instantly. He might have guessed who I was but would not have been able to confirm this until we were introduced. I hesitated for a while. It seemed a bit bizarre to sit there in a waiting room together, not speaking, when I knew he'd just been reading the intimate details of my life.

I decided that perhaps I ought to go and say hello, which took more guts than one might imagine. Taking the initiative to go and introduce yourself to a member of the peerage who you have only ever seen on the TV didn't come naturally to me.

I felt more like 13 than 30 as I walked up to him and extended my hand, 'Lord Winston, I'm Diane Blood. I have the advantage over you. I know who you are already because I have seen you on the television.'

He'd been reading a paper and for a second he seemed slightly taken aback. With the benefit of hindsight, I would say that this was just because he is an incredibly modest man, but at the time I didn't know if I'd done the right thing in going up and speaking to him before I was spoken to. After a short pause, which seemed like an age, he returned a warm smile and then came over to be introduced to my father.

I asked if he had read my evidence. I can't remember his exact response, but he confirmed that he had read every word and expressed sympathy in some way that usually prompts from the recipient the semi-automatic response of 'Oh, don't worry about it. It really doesn't matter.'

Words similar to these almost dribbled out of my mouth, until it occurred to me that it was rather stupid to say everything was all right when clearly it wasn't, otherwise I wouldn't be needing his help.

'It reads like a good fiction story, doesn't it? It's a shame it's real life.' I couldn't think of what else to say. I thought that comparing it to a story might distance it a bit and make it slightly less embarrassing that we were really talking about me.

The conference was productive. It gave everyone a chance to ask questions and clear up all the queries. At the end of the meeting, I went off on a side track to ask Lord Winston's advice on one point that was still nagging me – publicity. Because Lord Winston had frequently found himself in the public eye and understood better than anyone the effect of ethical infertility debates hitting the headlines, I thought he might be able to offer a different perspective on this point. I was still frightened to death of the effect of an ill-informed or, even worse, a one-sided public relations battle. Lord Winston pointed out that the timing of my case coincided with the Labour Party's pre-election conference, so, with this in mind, he thought that it would only make the inside pages. Other than that, it still really boiled down to the same old advice. It's your life, so you have to make the decision what to do. For now, it was easy. No one knew. Unless they found out, I'd keep quiet.

Lord Winston went away, wrote his opinion and the evidence was submitted to court. In his view, in the circumstances of our particular case, the doctors were justified in acting in the best interests of their patient (my husband) and complying with his wishes. The HFEA's expert witness had seen no justification for taking my husband's sperm, as it was not a life-saving measure. Lord Winston thought that there were broader interests to be taken into account. He also rebutted her concerns about the 'welfare of a child born without a father'. He pointed out that the law dictated that this was for the treating clinic to look into and decide. For his own part, he simply stated that there was 'no good evidence' to support the view that children born in circumstances such as the one I was contemplating were at any particular disadvantage. 'Nearly all the evidence suggesting that children nurtured by a single parent are at risk comes from those dysfunctional "families" who are in very disadvantaged financial or social circumstances.' He saw no ethical problem with treating me either and described the HFEA's refusal to allow export as 'harsh and unjust'.

I was pleased with his view and thought that we just had to sit back and wait for the hearing. I was wrong: with only a few days to go, the phone call I had been dreading arrived. It was Thursday. My case was to commence the following Wednesday. I learnt from my legal team that they had been contacted by Joshua Rozenberg, the BBC's legal affairs reporter. Without consulting either myself or my legal team, the HFEA had issued them with a press statement about my case and they were offering me the opportunity to balance the argument with an interview.

'It's time to stop dithering. The news is out and you have to decide what to do – now,' I was told. I didn't have time to consult either my parents or Steph's, but in any event it wasn't their decision to make. It was so important that I had to decide for myself and for Steph without regard to how others might feel. If it went wrong, I couldn't blame them afterwards.

'OK. I'll do it. I'll come down to London tomorrow.' I asked my legal team to negotiate an embargo until as close to the hearing as we could get. If it hit the Sunday papers, apart from the increased audience, I knew the backlash would rage the following week, right when I didn't want it. I'd thought about it long and hard, but had not really been able to resolve how I would handle the situation I now found myself in. At the end of the day, it was a snap decision to tell my side of the story, made in awkward circumstances. Not quite blind panic because I'd argued all the different scenarios through in my head a thousand times, but, as I'd never come to any conclusions, it was panic nevertheless.

Lord Lester arranged an interview with Joshua Rozenberg and also, at my request, with Clare Dyer, the legal correspondent for *The Guardian*. Apparently, she had been asking around and was probably pretty close to finding the story for herself. From my point of view, I didn't want anyone to have an exclusive. They always create far more news and controversy. Also, I didn't think it would be a good idea to give only the soundbites needed for TV or radio news and then leave the papers clamouring around for what to write without having anything I could refer them to.

The deal was done that both would embargo the story until Monday morning. My first meeting was with Clare at the barristers' chambers. I felt absolutely awful because I had a streaming cold and I was petrified. She wanted me to tell her everything; I basically didn't really want to say anything. I just wanted to answer questions that might stop someone from getting it all wrong. Clare, of course, didn't really know where to begin.

'So tell me what happened?' was far too broad a starting point. This was asking for my life story and, at 30 years old, even if I'd wanted to give it, it would have taken far too long. When I'd first briefed the solicitors about the case, it had taken two days. I needed to be able to distil it down, give the relevant points, without leaving myself feeling too exposed. It was almost impossible to do, and I hated it. It was especially hard referring to my late husband by his full name, Stephen. To me he'd usually been just Steph, but it didn't feel right that a journalist should get close enough to call him by the shortened form. From then on, I developed a tendency to frequently identify him as 'my husband'. I was less likely to trip up and forget if I avoided his name altogether.

No sooner had I completed the interview than I regretted it, just because I felt so bad afterwards. I kept thinking about what I had said and then imagining our personal details strewn across the pages of a newspaper. I was afraid she might have misunderstood some of the points I had made and it had also brought back to me details about Steph's death that I would rather not have relived. There was to be no real respite, however, as I then had just a few hours before offering myself up again for slaughter in the afternoon, when I had my appointment with Joshua Rozenberg back at the same chambers.

Gaining strength for the fight

At the end of the day, these people certainly caused me no harm and they reported my story in a fair, honest and careful manner; but at the time, I felt like a cornered animal with nowhere to run. Joshua Rozenberg had been busy making calls to my solicitor all morning. He knew that reporting restrictions meant that they couldn't show my image, but they wanted to film me so they could show it in shadow. I refused, saying that it would make me look as though I was ashamed or couldn't be identified because I'd done something wrong. In my opinion, that kind of footage always brings to mind criminals or prostitutes. The message went back and was understood. The BBC promised not to show me in shadow, but they wanted to film me anyway, just for posterity or in case they could ever use it at a later date. No one else seemed to see any harm in this, but I sent back the message, a clear 'No'. If any cameras were there, I wouldn't be.

I don't honestly know what they'd have done with the footage if they'd got it. Maybe it would have been sold to the foreign news syndicates who were not bound by UK reporting restrictions, maybe they'd have shown me in shadow despite our agreement or maybe they would have done exactly what they said – just kept it in case I later didn't mind it being shown. Whatever the case, I could see lots of pitfalls and no benefits of giving myself more to worry about with the presence of cameras. I would allow audio recording equipment only, but, with the barrage of requests, I was beginning to get slightly concerned in case they ignored my wishes and sneaked the cameras in anyway.

My dad had travelled down to London with me, so we went down the road to a local hotel where there was a seating area in which we could sit and 'relax' with a cup of coffee before my next appointment. I was incredibly wound up. I was so mortified by the experience of the interview with Clare Dyer and all the requests about cameras that, despite having nowhere to run and hide, I almost did precisely that. The InterCity out of King's Cross was beckoning rather temptingly and I almost obeyed its call. In my more lucid moments that lunchtime, it did occur to me that perhaps seriously annoying the BBC by not turning up for an appointment was not good for media relations, but, at that moment, I really didn't fancy the alternative.

When we met up with my solicitor, Richard Stein, before my next interview, my father confessed that I'd almost done a runner.

Richard was extremely grateful that I hadn't. I wouldn't have made him look too good either.

We knew that Joshua Rozenberg was already waiting for us at the chambers. I would have been informed if there had been any cameras. It seemed that all was clear on the Western Front, so I went in and we were introduced. Joshua must have sensed how nervous and mistrustful I was, as he opened his jacket like a magician verifying the authenticity of his act. 'Look, no cameras, I promise.'

I allowed myself a slight nervous laugh and then asked to see the statement the HFEA had issued. I wasn't allowed the opportunity to read it all, but saw enough to convince me that the BBC were not lying to me. They had been given the story either by the HFEA or their lawyers.

Joshua Rozenberg was extremely nice and thoughtful, and I felt much easier about his interview than I had about the earlier one. He had already decided on a list of about five questions which he wished to ask and he went through them first before turning on the tape recorder. I wasn't given the opportunity to rehearse. I know from my own experience of directing 'vox pop'-style interviews that it simply doesn't work and the respondent sounds totally unnatural. However, I was given the chance to mentally prepare and for my solicitor to advise if there was anything I could not answer. The questions were cleared and the recorder was turned on. It took quite a while to do the interview, partly because there were some people digging up the road outside and we were trying to record in the gaps when they were quiet. In the end, we gave in to the competition and moved to another office away from the noise. My solicitor was interviewed as well as myself.

The last question put to me, and the one Joshua Rozenberg advised would be used for the TV news, was simple: 'Why are you going to court? Why is this so important to you?'

My response was that I didn't have a choice. 'I wanted a baby. The fact that I've got to go through court and the publicity and all the rest of it is not by my choice. Really, what it boils down to is me and my husband had a life planned. We'd decided exactly what we wanted. I know what his feelings were – and I lost my husband, and I lost a part of that life, but I didn't lose the ability to have his child. That is still there and that is what I'm fighting for – I want the rest of my life back.'

Gaining strength for the fight

With the audio interview in the can, I now felt very relieved and much better than I had after the morning session. We had a bit of a discussion about what to show visually whilst my voice was being played on the TV, with me again emphasising my dislike for silhouetted figures. I think we actually agreed on a picture of the High Court because we couldn't think of anything else, but in the end the BBC actually used some footage of a rolling tape recorder, which I thought was OK.

The only detail left now was to check where and when anything would be appearing. Joshua Rozenberg called Clare Dyer from the office in my presence. She said that, unless anything huge hit over the weekend, it would be on the front page, which came as a bit of a shock after Lord Winston's comments about the competition for news space with the election coming up. I'd imagined a nice little piece tucked somewhere on the inside pages. Joshua also wanted to check that *The Guardian* would not publish before Monday. It was all a bit tense, with them both saying they were trusting the other not to let anything out before the agreed time. I suddenly thought they'd forgotten about me in all this, so I felt compelled to interject that I was trusting them both. That seemed to end the discussion. We put a blanket on it until Monday.

CHAPTER 8

The High Court hearing

I shut all the curtains and covered the only remaining window on my back door with a towel before going to bed on Sunday night. I half imagined I'd wake up to discover the media already camped on my lawn by the morning.

Before getting dressed, I peered tentatively through the front bedroom curtains. I decided that I was reasonably safe. The world still looked pretty much the same as usual and the sky wasn't about to cave in. I tuned in to Radio 4 for the early-morning *Today* programme and all was peaceful and relatively quiet.

I listened to my interview on *Today* and thought my point came across OK, but it was like lighting a blue touchpaper. No sooner had it been on that programme than it seemed to spread like wildfire. I had radios set to different stations in every room in my home and the TV remote control poised so I could flick from one channel to the next. It seemed like my case was being reported everywhere – simultaneously. Dad came up with a copy of *The Guardian* that I'd asked him to buy from the newsagents for me. The story was on the front page, but I didn't get a chance to study it in detail because I was too busy running around the house trying not to miss anything. Experts were being wheeled out left, right and centre, all giving their various comments. I knew that what was said now was critical. Reportage sways opinion, but opinion dictates editorial policy. It's one of those chicken-and-egg situations, but once everyone has decided which way the argument is going that's it, it snowballs and it's very hard to change. That's why I'd been so afraid of the HFEA giving their side to the story without giving mine in parallel. It's not one of those instances when you can sit back, assess the effect and then do anything about it later.

By nine o'clock my phone was going mad and representatives from the local newspaper were trying to hammer down my back door because they, like many others, had recognised my situation and voice. I kept the curtains shut and the towel on the back-door window proved useful after all. I told the journalists to go away, but they were annoyingly persistent and spent a good amount of the day standing in my drive, shouting through a locked door.

Both my parents and Stephen's were too busy monitoring the TV themselves to be of much assistance to me with the local journalists. Their phones were jammed with calls from a few very close friends and relatives who had suddenly recognised my situation. Until then, they had told no one. I think it came as a relief to them to suddenly be able to talk. Like myself, they were caught up in the unfolding situation, and we were all too concerned about public and professional opinion for any of us to be much support to each other.

The nationals did not hound me at first. Instead, they concentrated on bombarding my solicitors, Leigh, Day and Co. Richard Stein was out for the day so Martin Day, one of the partners, suddenly had to deal with it all when he didn't know me and obviously was less familiar with the case than Richard. He was thrown in at the deep end. Even my QC was missing for the day, so Martin had no one to turn to and was trying to deal with everything himself.

Independent Television News (ITN) gave him a particularly hard time, seriously hassling him for an interview with Leigh, Day and Co., if he couldn't arrange one with myself. They argued that it was totally unfair that the BBC had an interview whilst they had nothing to put out. They were right. I could imagine the chaos my story had caused when it was first broadcast and they realised they knew nothing about it, but I actually thought they had been doing an admirable job of making news on the hoof. I was totally amazed at the speed with which current affairs footage could be compiled, so quick it was almost like an echo of the opposite channel.

Martin was listening to the blackmail first-hand. By the time it got to me, it was diluted somewhat. He argued the points he was being fed: 'We have to issue a press release or they'll turn against you . . . You have to let me do an interview for ITN or they'll only report the HFEA's side of the story.' Martin thought we should meet their requests, especially in light of the fact that the HFEA were giving interviews. I argued against him, although there was some logic to what he said. To be honest, I was so busy monitoring the news and getting worked up about it that I couldn't think straight if I tried, let alone write a press statement. Martin said he'd write a draft one and send it to me. I agreed, on the understanding that it would not be released without my authorisation.

It took him a while to write. Until he faxed me his draft, I was still dithering over what to do. When I read the statement, it took me about two seconds to decide. As Martin didn't know me, he'd written what he thought and not what I thought.

I made the call right away to give Martin the message that I had decided: 'No. Nothing else is to go out. No interview with ITN. Nothing.'

I couldn't have someone else do it for me. It didn't work and, for now, I'd given all that I could give. Martin called me back a few minutes later to say that actually, on reflection and having tried to write the statement, he agreed with me. For now, I'd said all that needed to be said and everyone would just have to be content with referring to *The Guardian* and the BBC for my point of view.

By teatime, my interview for the BBC had been edited differently and was going out on ITV and Sky anyway. My first thought was that the BBC must have sold it. Maybe they gave it away or perhaps they didn't have copyright over what I gave them and it was sampled by the other stations. I'm not really familiar with what happens in these situations. Whatever the case, it obviously didn't get transferred complete with the instructions about my distaste for illustrating me in silhouette. On the other channels I started out as a shadow with fairly short, neat permed hair, of average build, and by the end of the day had turned into a much leaner figure with a long ponytail. It was obvious that, as the day wore on, they were being filled in with details of what I really looked like. Those who knew me thought that the library silhouette image they finally settled on was actually me. Clearly it wasn't.

Once it became obvious that there was no swaying either me or my solicitors to give any additional information or interviews, the whole circus calmed down somewhat and everyone became a lot more reasonable. The editors' letters and the money offers came rolling in, but the emotional arm-twisting stopped and no one became vindictive in their reporting.

The money offers were not huge at first. Well, no, I suppose it depends what you're comparing it with. If you could turn the clock back so I was only comparing it to my former salary, then it might have seemed quite a lot, but not when I'd grown used to the bottom-line figures on my legal bills and the expenses I was incurring running up and down to London every five minutes.

Money was not an issue anyway, as my life wasn't for sale. I was pleased about the offers, however, because I had been told from the start by my first solicitors that I couldn't win a case where the opposition knew that all they had to do was keep it going long enough to run me out of money. Obviously, the HFEA didn't have concrete knowledge of the state of my finances, but they would have a fair idea how much I'd have spent on legal fees already, they could see that I only lived in a modest suburban bungalow and they would know that I couldn't really earn anything whilst I was tied up with the legal wrangle. As it was in evidence that I ran my own company, for a small fee they could even get details of my income from Companies House, should they ever get that curious. Now, with all the offers flooding in, I was an unknown quantity in financial terms.

What was most uplifting about the day, though, was suddenly discovering that I had supporters of whom I'd been unaware. I'd begun to feel that perhaps my close little team who were helping me with the legal case, the couple of clinics in the USA, the one in Greece and possibly the one in Belgium, were the only people who agreed with my point of view. Now there were people on television, people I could never have found even if I had dared to ask. Some were for me, some were against. Those who attacked me tore at my heart, but everyone who spoke in my favour was a revelation. Most surprising of all was the support of Baroness Warnock.

In 1982, Baroness Warnock had chaired the Committee of Inquiry into Human Fertilisation and Embryology. Their report in 1984 claimed they had 'grave misgivings' about posthumous artificial insemination by husband. They felt it 'may give rise to profound psychological problems for the child and the mother'. The HFEA had submitted evidence from both this report and the government White Paper produced following it, which reinforced that the committee had felt that posthumous conception should be 'actively discouraged'. Yet here was Mary Warnock herself, on the television saying that personally she hoped I would be allowed to have my baby. The legal team, my parents, everyone must have been watching, as we were all on the phone to one another within seconds.

'Baroness Warnock is on the telly. Can we get a statement from her for court evidence?'

My solicitor got to work on it and we got our statement, which was submitted into evidence at the eleventh hour. This was important, as she was able to explain to the court that she felt 'certain that had the Committee of Inquiry considered such a case [as mine] we would have seen no ethical or public policy objections to allowing the woman to become pregnant by the use of her husband's frozen sperm, either in this country or abroad, given the particular facts'.

Also at this very late stage we learnt, almost by accident, on rereading a letter from Professor Cooke from the Sheffield clinic on another matter, that the Belgian clinic at some point in the past had come back to him and told him that their ethics committee had agreed to treat me. It was there in black and white, but we hadn't picked up on it because it was squeezed in between a whole load of other details. There was no time to get a letter from the clinic themselves, so we rang Professor Cooke to double-check the facts and asked him to put it down in a separate letter, which he managed to turn around extremely quickly. We switched tack from Greece to Belgium and submitted Professor Cooke's letter into evidence.

We were on a high and ready to go. The adrenalin rush felt good and probably prevented me from cracking up completely at a time I had envisaged would be almost impossible to live through.

I made most of the front pages on Tuesday morning, but I didn't read them. There was no point. It was too late to do anything about it anyway, even if they had been full of inaccuracies. We spent Tuesday travelling down to London by car and we would be in court on Wednesday morning. The judge would soon be able to hear my story for himself. There wasn't time to be prejudiced by the media.

The High Court hearing

My parents and I stayed in a central London hotel. Stephen's parents travelled down separately and stayed with Steph's sister and brother-in-law on the outskirts of London. They were all coming to the hearing. We knew there would be a herd of photographers waiting outside the court, so we decided to meet up inside the building to avoid some of the problems that created. Even though I still had an order preventing my image from being published, there was nothing to stop them photographing my relatives and identifying me by association. I didn't know how my relatives felt about the possibility of their photographs being published, but I was aware of the impact that the case was having on their lives as well as my own.

My parents and I had a big discussion the night before about which entrance to use to the High Court. There are actually loads of ways in and out, so no one really needs to run the gauntlet of photographers if they don't want to. You can always use a back entrance. The photographers cannot possibly cover them all and do not try.

Now, you might think that the decision would be simple. If you don't want to face the pack, just sneak in the back door. But it was much more complicated than that for me. I believed that justice would be done. I revered the High Court and I needed to feel that I had been there. Also, running in through the tradesmen's entrance had the overtones of someone who was ashamed or had something to hide. I decided to take a deep breath and walk through the middle of them all with my head held high; albeit with the knowledge that they could not print my picture in any British publication after they had busied themselves taking it.

When we met up inside the High Court on the Wednesday morning, the mood was still quite buoyant. Mike Fordham, my barrister, came across to inform me that a Teletext opinion poll had closed that morning with 90 per cent of the public in my favour. I hadn't really known which way the opinion was falling because I'd stopped looking at the reports, so I was overjoyed. That was a pretty massive majority, so I felt I no longer needed to get so uptight about the damning negative views that I knew were still being expressed. I'm not saying they didn't hurt on an emotional level because they did – bitterly. But intellectually I am aware that once people have made up their mind, they stop listening and a 90 per cent majority is very hard to change.

Of course, I still had to face the judgement of the court, which was all-important and quite a separate issue from that of the public, although in a way public opinion did make a slight difference to the case because our argument for export under EC law relied on the HFEA not being able to claim they were protecting a public policy, such as defending society from an erosion of moral or ethical values. They claimed there was such a defence, although they never explicitly stated what it was. We said there wasn't. Had 90 per cent of the public supported their stance and not mine, I think they might have had a point, but I can't see how you can defend a public policy for a point of law that the vast majority of the public disagree with. Probably more importantly than that, it made a difference to me. Whilst I had accepted it, I had dreaded the possibility of living the rest of my life thinking that everyone hated me.

That morning I also received the first of many letters I was to get from members of the public. It had arrived at my solicitor's, so he had brought it to court with him to give to me. It was from a woman who thanked me for taking the issue to court. She said that she had discussed my case with her husband and knew that if he was to die suddenly before they were able to have a child, they would still want her to have the opportunity to try for that child after his death. It was rather touching, but I felt a bit of a fraud living with her gratitude because I hadn't gone to court to uphold a principle or for the benefit of anyone else. I'm not saying that now I thought about it I didn't hope that what I was doing might potentially help this woman, her partner and others like them, but I'd been rather selfish. I was going to court for my husband and myself. Had there been any other option, I would have gladly taken it.

Like the preliminary hearing, the case was brought before Sir Stephen Brown, President of the Family Division. It was held in the same courtroom, with its austere dark wooden panelling and pew-like benches. My father and I sat right at the very front with Richard, my solicitor. We were positioned in the middle on the row in front of the QCs. All the Counsel knew each other because they worked in the same chambers, which at first seemed a bit bizarre, although it actually also made things far simpler because they could liaise with each other easily to arrange court dates and other matters.

The High Court hearing

Lord Lester, my QC, was behind me on the left. David Pannick leaned over to introduce himself to me as the HFEA's QC, behind me to my right. Behind the QCs were their respective junior Counsel, Michael Fordham and Dinah Rose. Behind Dinah Rose, the HFEA's barrister, were their solicitors, and, right at the very back of the court, there was the public gallery. My mother sat with Stephen's family and some of his former work colleagues somewhere between the legal people and the rest of the public. In front of me, to my right and at right angles to the judge's bench and the rest of the seating, were the benches packed with reporters. I don't know where the representatives from the HFEA were because I found it hard and a bit impolite to look. I didn't really have a problem with David Pannick because he'd introduced himself, but when I'd briefly made eye contact with Dinah Rose outside the court, our eyes had danced apart as though charged with a sudden shock of electricity. I hadn't intended it to happen. I don't suppose she did either, if she noticed. I was actually looking at her not because I knew she was on the opposing team but because she was wearing a shorter version of the coat I had on. I was rather embarrassed by the involuntary reaction and it wasn't an experience I wished to repeat.

I knew that everyone was just doing their jobs and I tried desperately hard not to take anything personally, but to me it was far more than a job. It was my life. When I wasn't praying for justice, I found myself confessing to having feelings of bitterness towards those who spoke against me, and I prayed very hard for the grace to accept and forgive the intrusion into my life. I was actually very glad that the HFEA, like me, had a good legal team. It gets everything clear right from the start. There was no mix-up and everyone gave it their best shot. It made things better for me, as well as for them. The court and publicity ordeal was not an experience I would wish to relive, but I don't find myself wishing everything had been easy and it had never happened. Indeed, there were incredibly heartening moments that I would not wish to forget, although I hope that neither myself nor anyone else will ever have to go through anything like it again.

Sitting through the three days of the first court hearing was not pleasant. Nobody was forcing me to be there, but I would have been equally anxious if I had been some place else. There was no escape and in any event I needed to know the details. I could not have lived with myself afterwards if I had not known what was going on.

The first day was the easiest, and I was particularly grateful that Lord Winston made it to hear the proceedings, even though he was forced to arrive a little late. Someone handed me a piece of paper to inform me when he entered the court. He'd been at the Labour Party conference in Blackpool and had got up at 4 a.m. just to drive back to London and be there.

Our side went first and my QC spoke for the whole day. I'd heard it all before and had had to become as hardened as humanly possible to reliving the distressing details of Stephen's death. It was his family I felt for. I had been over and over it a thousand times, checking every last detail, making sure it was correct. They hadn't. I hadn't wanted to hurt them, but now I had no choice. I'd given them the opening statement to read shortly before the hearing, but giving it the once-over is not the same as hearing it in court in front of strangers. I know they found it particularly harrowing.

The opening statement dealt with the facts, then we moved on to the legal propositions. We argued down three routes. The first would have given me the right to ask for treatment in the UK; the other two alternatives would have afforded me the opportunity to have treatment abroad. Winning on any one of them would have been a victory. I did not mind where I was treated. I would have taken any path open to me.

The 1990 Act was primarily concerned with protecting third-party donors. It was not meant to legislate between husbands and wives, as it excluded those who were being 'treated together'. We actually took this to mean married or cohabiting couples, but later discovered that it even covers situations where a man has agreed to donate his sperm with the intention of helping a female friend, for example in a situation where her partner was infertile. The sperm donor need not be her lover.

According to the HFEA's interpretation of the Act, my husband's death turned him into someone with whom I had no more connection than an anonymous donor. To my way of thinking, this had to be wrong. For treatment in the UK, we argued that my husband's death did not turn him into a third-party donor and that we could still be 'treated together', and therefore be excluded from the Act, even though he had died after the samples were taken. We argued that his treatment was the removal of the sperm. At that point we were 'together'. He was alive. Therefore he was still my husband and did not have to provide written consent. My husband's physical presence at my treatment was no more a necessity than it would have been had he still been alive.

On treatment abroad, we covered two points. My rights to unimpaired access to the medical treatment I desired in another member state of the European Union and how reasonable the HFEA's decisions were in light of their acknowledged discretionary powers.

The Authority had the discretion to allow me to export Stephen's sperm despite any domestic restrictions. They just decided not to. This one really hurt. I felt the circumstances of my case were very individual and important. In light of the fact that they had made up their minds without any knowlededge of our particular situation, before we went to court we had asked them to reconsider and take my evidence into account once it was available. They had declined on the grounds that the individual circumstances were irrelevant to their decision.

I so desperately wanted to speak to these people face to face. I couldn't understand how they could make decisions about my life without meeting me and giving me the opportunity to answer their questions. It was incredibly frustrating. I felt as though I was being kept at arm's length, so they didn't have to see me as a real person. I began to feel as though I was actually being viewed as the silhouette portrayal shown on Independent Television News, a symbolic outline with no inner feelings. From the Authority's point of view, I could see the benefit of maintaining emotional detachment, but when deciding about an emotional issue, it seemed to me an impossible and unbelievably cruel stance.

At least the judge got to hear my side of the story and ask questions. Of course, he still couldn't ask me first-hand. Quite apart from the fact that I would have been incapable of explaining the legal issues, even on a personal level everything was still probably put far more eloquently though my QC than I could ever have been capable of. However, it didn't stop the judge from staring straight into my eyes, as though trying to read my soul, when waiting for the response to many pertinent and personal questions. He asked for a few clarifications about our relationship and beliefs, and about the events surrounding Stephen's death. Sometimes he expected a response from Lord Lester, but at other points it was more that he was making a comment. I stared back, hoping he could see the answers, and occasionally I allowed myself a nervous little smile. The strain of involuntary emotional expression made my facial muscles ache. By the end of the day I was as exhausted as if I'd been doing all the talking, and I hadn't said a word. I found myself anxiously watching the clock tick out the remaining minutes.

I left the courtroom with a certain amount of relief that the first day was over. I didn't think it had gone as well as it could have, as the judge hadn't seemed to either agree with or grasp all of our arguments. Neither did I feel that it had been a total disaster, though, as he also appeared sympathetic to my plight.

My party almost left the High Court by a rear entrance, but then we decided to go back in and leave by the front door, just to show that I was not ashamed and was not about to crawl away and give in quietly. It was a bit strange really, because we'd actually been outside once and not seen a single photographer, but when we went out the front door there were hordes of them and they must have been waiting for ages because it had taken us such a long time to get there. It made me wonder how long they would have waited in vain if we had left via the back door.

I didn't really think it had gone well enough for a broad grin, but I certainly didn't wish the headlines to tell the judge or the HFEA of my fears, so I obliged the photographers and smiled. I might have found this a little hard, but I was aided somewhat by Lord Lester, my QC, who was following a few paces behind me. We couldn't have a sensible conversation with all the reporters and photographers listening, so he was telling me that it was my tenth birthday and I was very happy because I'd just come downstairs to find a room full of lovely presents waiting for me. I wasn't too good at imagining the presents but, after a rather tense day in court, the ridiculousness of such trivial banter and the photographers snapping away, running backwards in front of me, as though their life depended on it, was rather amusing.

Judging from their accents, many of the photographers waiting for me on that first day were American. My lawyers had warned me that the photographers would still be able to sell my image overseas, and I imagined they must be working for US publications. One of them eventually pleaded with me to stop walking just long enough for them to get a decent shot so he could go home, stop worrying and feed the kids for a bit longer. I stopped. Photographers are often portrayed as heartless hunters. It comes as quite a jolt to realise that maybe they're just trying to survive like the rest of us.

Day two in court commenced with the brief completion of our submissions and then moved on to the case for the HFEA. I didn't expect the day to be a happy experience, and it wasn't. I watched every second tick by on the clock, praying that it would soon be over and it would be our turn to answer back. Initially, the hearing had been scheduled for just two days, but because we had been so concerned to make sure the judge understood our points, Lord Lester had taken a little longer than envisaged. We had therefore expected David Pannick, QC for the HFEA, to talk for the rest of the day, but he threw us by finishing early. He made his points quickly and succinctly. He could do this because it was obvious that the judge was taking on board what he said.

David Pannick made it all sound so plausible and logical. Written consent for storage was mandatory and there was no way round it. Unless we were being 'treated together', the same was true for treatment. We couldn't be treated together as my husband was dead. As regards export, the Authority had decided not to depart from the principle in their general directions. It was their choice. The HFEA required written consent for export and believed it should not be used as a way of evading domestic law. In short, if a UK citizen cannot have treatment in the UK, she should not therefore be permitted to have it elsewhere. These matters had been debated by Parliament and were a matter of social and public policy. In relation to EC law, I was not being denied freedom of access to treatment. I could have treatment with sperm which was available in another EU member state, but I couldn't take my husband's sperm with me.

Every point raised against me felt like a body blow and if the judge made expressions of sympathy with the HFEA's argument, it hurt all the more. My heart was on the floor and when Lord Lester had to get back on his feet again, we all felt as though he was fighting a lost cause. We needed time to rally our defences and, cleverly, David Pannick had left us with barely enough time, but sufficient to put us under pressure to finish that day. I was immensely grateful when Lord Lester managed to talk out the rest of the day without the judge putting us under too much duress to finish quickly.

I believed that I had lost. It seemed obvious to me from the comments that the judge was making, but it still came as a shock when Lord Lester and Michael Fordham called a quick team briefing around the table outside the courtroom to confirm that this was also their experienced view. Lord Lester told me, 'This judge has stopped listening.'

We were all present – my entire legal team, my parents, Stephen's parents, his sister and brother-in-law. Everyone else was thunderstruck. It seemed that my family had not picked up on the subtle nuances that both my legal team and I had sensed.

Lord Lester needed to know whether I would wish to appeal, as it would affect the way they would close their submissions. If I didn't want to appeal, they would sum up quickly and stop wasting everybody's time. It was an awful decision to have to make and I suspect an even worse question to have to ask.

I didn't want to give up, but I knew that everyone else was tired. I really didn't want to have to drag them through it all again. I believed at that moment that if I could have resigned myself to walk away, it would have made my family happy. They too could have rested knowing that I had tried. They would have been unhappy that I had lost, but I think that at that point they saw it as a preferable option to running up more bills, rubbing salt into raw wounds and going through the ordeal all over again. There was only one problem with this theory. I couldn't say I could walk away. I voiced my concerns about their feelings, particularly those of Stephen's parents, as did Michael Fordham, my barrister. We asked for their contributions to the debate, but, basically, everyone thought that only I could make the decision.

I didn't know where I was going to get the money from to continue on to an appeal. Selling out to the newspapers was always an option, but not a very attractive one. Besides, although it would provide a huge lump sum, there was no guarantee it would be enough to get to the end. Running out of money halfway through was no use to anyone. There was no point getting emotionally exhausted over something I didn't have the resources to finish.

To be honest, my side were already working at reduced costs and I don't think they'd have hung up their wigs and gowns if I'd have been able to pay them nothing. My constant fear was ending up with the costs being awarded against me from the other side if I lost. I was already looking at a probable £30,000 for the HFEA's legal fees from this hearing alone. I was earning nothing and living on food hand-outs from my parents. I couldn't see any way out.

My legal team left. Lord Lester and Michael Fordham needed to go back to chambers and prepare for the following day. I promised to phone them with my decision, but I guess I'd already said enough for them to know what it was. By the time I called, they'd already worked on the assumption that I would appeal. They had rallied their own arguments against David Pannick QC. The writing was on the wall that we were going to lose, but they weren't giving in yet. They were still going to give it their all and try to persude Sir Stephen Brown. In Michael's own words, 'We're going down fighting.'

As for the rest of us, we'd hung around in the court for a while, discussing things between ourselves. Stephen's former work colleagues who were there with us were particularly concerned that I shouldn't make the decision on financial grounds. They said I should just trust that the money would come from somewhere. Stephen's family asked if I'd mind if they didn't come back to court on the last day. They didn't want to see us beaten into the ground and they didn't want to face the media yet again. In a way, I was relieved that they'd opted out because I didn't want to feel responsible for their own emotions as well as my own.

I left by the front door to the High Court. The photographers were still outside, not as many as the day before, but they were obviously pretty persistent to wait so long. I smiled and made a quick retreat back to the hotel, where I called Counsel's chambers to deliver the news that they already knew. 'I want to appeal.'

God willing, I'd take it all the way to Europe if I had to. Having examined my emotions in the face of failure, I now knew that it was futile even pretending to consider that I could give up at any stage. For me, it just wasn't an option.

In the end, it was rather a shame that Stephen's family didn't come back to court on the last day. I later learnt that they almost changed their mind and came, but, having told me they wouldn't, they eventually decided to stick with what we had agreed. I was sad they didn't come because it was rather uplifting and, in my view, the best day of the three. Our counter-arguments sounded convincing. Lord Lester explained why our interpretation of the law made more sense than the HFEA's, and the judge appeared refreshed and more attentive. Michael Fordham and Lord Lester must have been working half the night. They really tried to turn the case around and, at lunchtime, when it was all over, I left thinking that I still had a chance of Sir Stephen Brown deciding in my favour.

CHAPTER 9

High Court judgement

Hoping for the best, yet fearing the worst, I dreaded going back home after the court case. I vaguely imagined that walking back into my little bungalow for the first time might be as bad as when I first went back after my husband had died. I thought it would be cold and uninviting, as it had felt on that occasion.

Not so. Instead I was greeted by a pile of letters waiting for me on my doormat. Some were from former friends or work colleagues whom I had long since lost touch with. They had deduced my identity and wished to offer me their support. Others were from total strangers. One of these was pretty vitriolic, but the kind wishes contained in all the rest cheered me up no end. Above all else, I was incredibly relieved that I no longer had to hide or deceive people. I found a certain amount of peace in having finally 'come out' and said, 'This is me. This is what my husband and I believed in and what I will fight for.' Whether people agreed or disagreed was relatively immaterial. I was just so grateful that I no longer had to live a lie. I could be myself and, to a degree, the identity that I had lost with the initial refusal of the HFEA to allow me to carry out my own and my late husband's wishes was reinstated. I had a voice and people cared enough to listen. My friends understood why I had not confided in them and tried to offer support.

Steph's mum and dad invited me up for Sunday lunch at the weekend. We had a really good chat and I was surprised to find that they too had been very strained by the pressure of keeping silent. I think the ability to speak openly and freely, and also for our friends to approach us, was a great relief to us all. Without it, I'm not sure if any of us could have gone on. To me, it was like I had found my second wind and Steph's parents also seemed to have been lifted after the oppressive court atmosphere. They were brilliant, offering me their understanding and support as we talked about strategy for continuing to appeal. Of course, I also told them about the last day in court and we all hoped that further action wouldn't be necessary.

The pressure was now on to go out and earn some money. Although emotionally I wasn't particularly well equipped for committing fully to work, I didn't have an endless reserve of savings to draw on. The Baby and Child Show at Earls Court commenced just a couple of days after my court case ended. Baby and Child is one of only two major nursery shows a year and, as usual, Clippasafe, my client whose business I'd resigned in January, were exhibiting. I'd gone to the show every year for as long as I could remember. To be honest, if you're going to work for anyone in an industry, particularly on the promotion side, visiting the trade exhibitions is central to your understanding of the market and competition. It is also the ideal opportunity to renew and refresh links with the various specialist press reporters – essential for pitching and targeting PR.

If I was going to start work seriously again, I needed to go to the exhibition, although walking into a large hall full of baby products was not a thought I relished. In the end, I didn't really have a choice. It wasn't just the money; I also couldn't afford to become too insulated and I needed the outside contact yielded by work.

I took a deep breath, held my head up high and wandered in. The initial shock of hubbub and baby paraphernalia was rather like inadvertently charging into a brick wall; but once I'd stood there for a while, I realised that the wall was only of as much substance as I allowed it to be. I walked right through it and appeared out the other side, relatively unscathed.

I didn't stay at the exhibition long, but I did go and visit Clippasafe. They now understood, for the first time, my reasons for resigning their PR business at the beginning of the year. They sympathised and were generally very understanding. Fortunately for me, they had not yet found a replacement for my company. I explained that I thought I would probably lose the court case but that I wished to appeal and I was looking to start doing some work again. It was great just to be able to lay my cards on the table and review the situation openly and honestly. We agreed to reinstate our former working relationship as from that month.

I found it quite ironic that, although I had been so fearful of the news of my situation breaking, it had actually given back to me two important elements of my life. First, it had given me back my friends. Now, my work. It was just a shame that the remaining missing chunk looked set to prove so elusive. The part of my life I desired the most was to be able to carry on and have our child. If only the court would come back with a positive answer, the world would be full of sunshine and roses once more.

Time moved on and there was still no news of an impending judgement. I'd expected it to come pretty quickly, because I believed the judge had made up his mind in those first couple of days of the hearing. If he was going to rule against me, I didn't see why he needed any longer to think about it. The longer it took to announce the judgement, therefore, the more hopeful I became. I thought that the final day in court might have made some impact after all, and I really began to think the outcome would be the one I was looking for. Also, the longer the memory of those awful first two days in court dimmed into the past, the more our expectations were raised. After all, to me, our arguments made far more sense than the HFEA's, so it was pretty hard to continue to bear their view in mind.

Some of Stephen's friends and former colleagues had begun to work on the Stephen Blood Baby Appeal, a trust aimed at raising awareness and money to help me continue with the court battle if I should lose this first hearing. They were determined that Stephen's wishes shouldn't be undermined for want of cash and also that the same thing should not happen to anyone else.

It was a difficult balancing act because their proposals themselves would have a price. Phone lines and a bank account would need to be set up and the discretionary trust fund itself would have to be drawn up by a solicitor. Also, they would need to hire rooms for press conferences to publicise the fund and the issue my case had raised. The proposed trustees ended up being the instigators, the bank manager and a solicitor. Some of my former colleagues got roped in too. A logo was designed and an advertising agency produced artwork ready to output as posters, if they should be needed. Everything was in place and ready to go at the touch of a button, but we all hoped and prayed it wouldn't be needed.

Stephen's friends who were busy doing all this were very well meaning, but I was still a bit unsure. They knew absolutely nothing about PR and I didn't think they realised quite what they were getting themselves into. Besides which, if it was going to work at all, I knew it would be me who would have to do 90 per cent of the talking at press conferences, and I wasn't exactly an expert on that front either. Pumping out banal press releases and a spot of minor crisis management for a consumer watchdog programme was the closest my PR experience had ever led me to handling such a situation. It wasn't quite in the same league. I knew there was much I needed to learn but didn't know exactly what.

If Stephen's friends were going to go through with their plans (to be honest, even if they weren't) with the current interest in my case, we all needed some first-class media training. If I lost, I could request that the anonymity order be lifted, but, given the judge's feelings on the subject, with no possibility even of a child to protect, it was a realistic possibility that it would be lifted anyway, irrespective of my wishes.

We called the chairman of NABS, the National Advertising and Benevolent Society, a charity funded by and aimed at helping people who work in advertising. They could help, but it was going to cost a small fortune for advice. Not much use really and not very charitable. Next I called some people I used to go to college with who worked in a top London agency. They and their manager were much more helpful, but we eventually ended up sitting in the London office of Jane Atkinson, the former press relations manager to the Princess of Wales. Her advice came pro bono. I went down to see her with my father and Paul Plant, who had appointed himself the main spokesperson for the Stephen Blood Baby Appeal. It was just a couple of days before the judgement was finally delivered. Jane's advice was that Paul and I needed media training – fast – and she managed to organise a two-hour session for the next day. My solicitors had a scrapbook full of press clippings to date, so we couriered it round to the media trainers to allow them to prepare.

I'm not really sure what I learnt. Most of it probably went straight out the window the instant someone shoved a microphone under my nose, but I do know it was useful practice. We worked on the principle that I was going to lose. If I won, it didn't really matter what the media said or did.

Before the training, I'd had some vague notion that I was going to get out of the court without speaking to anyone and we could then have a nice little press conference some time later. They told us that this was unrealistic, so we practised walking out of a building with people firing questions at us and jostling us with video cameras. We decided just to give a quick 'soundbite' and then invite the journalists to a press conference later. I soon discovered how incredibly difficult it is not to answer a question when someone addresses you directly; my parents must have done a reasonable job of bringing me up. Everyone knows that if someone speaks to you, it is impolite not to answer. Responding is almost instinctive. It's certainly not something you can 'unlearn' in two hours, although it was useful to be made aware of how easy it would have been to spill the whole story whilst standing on the court steps.

Other than that, Paul and I were taught to speak in short sentences, to answer a question and then stop, rather than keep going over the same point. Unlike Paul, who plays a good Widow Twanky at his kids' Christmas pantomimes and was probably more used to taking centre stage, I was incredibly nervous to be on the wrong side of a camera. During the course of my career, I've directed many photo shoots and videos, but telling someone else what to do is not the same as doing it yourself. The training helped prepare me.

Part of the way through the session, I received a phone call from my solicitor's secretary, Shirley. She had called to give me the time of the judgement. It was to be given the following day. When I knew who it was, I hardly dared take the call. I knew that by now my solicitors would know the judgement, even though they couldn't tell me until an hour before it was given out in court. Shirley sounded downbeat. I knew I'd lost.

Even harder than taking the phone call was walking back into the media training room, knowing that it was all needed and tomorrow it would be for real. My parents, who'd been sitting on the sidelines watching us, looked anxiously at me. I told them the time of the judgement. I wanted to have a break to cry, but we were on limited time, so instead I just said, 'I think we'd better continue. I get the feeling it's not good news.' The hugs and sympathy were saved for later. For now, it was back to work. I wasn't going to be beaten and I knew that if, mentally, I caved in, that was precisely what would happen.

Despite some attempts at rationalising that my guess was probably entirely wrong, decisions had to be made, working on the premise that I'd lost. We decided to book a room for a press conference at the Waldorf, as it was a good central location and, at that point, it was the only place we knew of. We put out an invitation on the Press Association wires that night. We also issued instructions to my solicitors that, if my suspicions were correct, I was still determined to appeal and I wished to drop anonymity. I'd come to the conclusion that it was a bit of a farce anyway, as most of the papers knew who I was. One had even obtained a copy of Stephen's obituary from my local paper and contacted all the mourners to see what they could uncover. With everyone else speaking to the newspapers, I decided that perhaps I was better off doing the talking for myself. I feared that if I left the order in place, anonymity might yet become a hindrance.

If this sounds terribly organised, I can assure you it wasn't. It was all rather hurried and there were some things I just didn't consider at all. For instance, I was trying to avoid any papers getting exclusive rights to photographs of Stephen and myself. A wedding photographer in Worksop apparently genuinely thought he had taken our photos when he'd been approached by one newspaper. Allegedly he'd been offered £10,000 for the exclusive rights to print them. Fortunately for me, he hadn't even been at my wedding and as my real wedding photographer was actually based in Nottingham, I didn't think any of the papers would find him. I hadn't thought to contact him and organise a considered plan of action.

At the eleventh hour, I ended up dragging some friends up from Grantham to babysit my bungalow. I'd temporarily taken down my framed photographs, so nothing could be photographed through any of the windows, but I didn't really like the idea of journalists, or anyone else for that matter, snooping around when no one was at home. When most people go away for a few days, they don't find it broadcast on *News at Ten*. Again, I just didn't think about this until it was almost too late.

Meanwhile, the money offers now rolling in from the newspapers were doubling by the second. As I mentioned before, the figures hadn't really started out that high, but with them all wondering why I wasn't selling and fearing that someone else would get the story, it seemed that they all had instructions to buy at any price. You could almost taste their panic.

You see, for newspapers, buying a single story is never going to increase their readership by enough to justify the money it costs. As I understand it, it is all about kudos and making sure that your competition doesn't get something that you don't have. It was amusing, flattering but, above all else, frightening. I was turning down sums of money that were almost beyond my imagination. Several people pointed out that I must be mad. But the money wasn't remotely important, except for the fact that I desperately needed it to continue the court case. I tried to trust that God would provide for my needs, but it wasn't easy. I was worried in case I later discovered I couldn't raise the cash by any other means.

The other factor which discouraged me from selling my story was that I knew that the newspapers who hadn't struck the deal would probably do their best to discredit my case. One gets the exclusive rights and has access to the correct details and reasoning, the other seven major English nationals would all have to make up their own version and try to make the story that their competitor had secured appear worthless. Besides that, I didn't want to give a newspaper access to my story for the rest of my life. Who could tell at that stage how long it would all continue for?

Once I had walked into my planned press conference and spilt the beans, my story would be relatively worthless in financial terms. I was acutely aware of this and I didn't really need the various editors to keep pointing it out. Obviously, they felt they needed to, just to keep screwing down the pressure. Finally, I almost blew my resolve not to give an exclusive. I instructed my solicitor (who was currently turning down all the offers on my behalf) that I might consider a deal from anyone who was prepared to fund my fees and any costs awarded against me, after taxation, to appeal. This would mean it could cost them nothing if I won or an unquantifiable amount if I lost. Basically, I wanted someone to take on part of the risk that I was currently facing. Even though, in the worst case scenario, it would probably be far less than the current bidding, this one threw them completely. It seemed that no one had the faith to take a gamble. Their response was just to offer more money as a fixed sum. I wasn't interested and I told my solicitors and my parents, who were doing the liaising for me, that I no longer wanted to hear the amounts. I didn't see any point in getting myself stressed out by it any longer. The final figures of which I was aware just before entering court were around the £110,000 mark. The last thing I heard before walking in was, 'Whatever you've been offered, I've been authorised to double it.' It could have been Mickey Mouse speaking, for all I knew. It was all rather silly, but I suppose to them it was serious business.

For me, the only serious business was the legal proceedings. I'd been called to my QC and barrister's chambers just before the judgement. I was accompanied by my parents and Neil, another friend of Stephen's from the Stephen Blood Baby Appeal. He was going to stay with my mum and help her through the crowds of reporters if things got a bit frantic, leaving my dad to look after me. The meeting at chambers was for a final discussion and to give my legal team their instructions once I had been made aware of the ruling. They handed me the document to read. It was, as I expected, full of sympathy, but nothing of any use. Sure enough, I'd lost. We were bitterly disappointed, but it came as no great surprise to any of us.

Sir Stephen Brown had been persuaded by David Pannick's arguments on EC law and agreed that it was impossible for my husband and me to be regarded as being 'treated together' as Stephen was no longer here and had been unconscious when the treatment began. He concluded his judgement by saying that Parliament had entrusted the responsibility for decisions on 'the fundamental matter in question', which I assume meant export, to the Human Fertilisation and Embryology Authority. The court could only see whether the Authority had acted properly within the scope of its discretion and it didn't assist me 'for the Court to express the view that it might itself have made a different decision if it had the authority to do so'. The decision rested with the HFEA. They could decide to allow export, but hadn't. The Court implied it would have allowed export, but the judge was right, knowing that didn't help me one little bit. I felt as though I had been mortally wounded and this was like rubbing salt into it. Everyone wanted to wash their hands of my problem. My life blood seemed to be ebbing away and no one wanted to bear the stain. The HFEA blamed the law. The court blamed Parliament and the HFEA. All I could do was reaffirm my desire to appeal and to drop anonymity.

'There is just one thing I have to put to you,' my QC said. 'The other side have said that if you don't appeal, they will not ask for their costs.'

I knew that this would amount to somewhere in the region of £30,000. I felt hurt and insulted. To me, this seemed tantamount to blackmail.

'It still doesn't matter, I want to appeal. How could they think that costs could matter in something like this?' They obviously didn't have a clue how strongly I felt about the issue to come up with something like that.

Lord Lester felt that perhaps he ought to check that my understanding of the offer was correct, so he rang to speak to the HFEA's barrister. 'I just want to check the terms of this offer regarding appeal. Is the position that you will not press for costs if my client is refused leave to appeal, even if she asks for it, or is it that we must not ask to appeal?'

The answer was obviously that I mustn't ask and that they would be opposing my request.

Lord Lester continued, 'Ah, well, in that case I feel I must advise the judge about this. We will be requesting leave to appeal.'

Apparently, at that point, the HFEA's barrister said the offer was made 'without prejudice', so Lord Lester did not tell the judge.

No matter what fancy phrase was attached to the offer, which at the time I didn't really understand anyway, it still felt like a kind of bribery and potentially a rather strange perversion of the course of justice.

The discussion over with, we walked across the road to the court, quickly wading our way through the microphones and reporters. 'Are you going to drop anonymity? Will you appeal if you lose? How will you celebrate if you win?'

'You'll have to wait and see. Please come to my press conference afterwards,' was about all I could manage as I rushed past.

We were running late, so we couldn't have hung about to answer their questions even if I'd wanted to. Worse than that, perhaps it was nerves, or perhaps it was just that I'd been chasing around like an idiot all morning and hadn't had time to go, but I really needed the loo. I thought that perhaps I'd get a chance to go once we were in the court building, but a quick look at my watch confirmed that there simply wasn't time.

We went into court and rose for the judge to enter. He read through the judgement, I suppose for the benefit of the reporters and other interested members of the public who'd come to hear it. Of course, I'd just read it before we went into court, so I didn't have to listen too hard to take it in. This was just as well, because I don't think I could have concentrated. I was far too desperate to answer the call of nature. I finally realised that I simply wasn't going to last out to the end of the session, and I really didn't want to miss the request for appeal. I looked at my dad and scrawled on my judgement paper that I needed to go to the toilet. Dad replied back by writing a single word, 'Go.'

I virtually ran out of the courtroom. My mum, who was sitting with Neil nearer the back of the court, followed me to see if I was all right and the reporters all followed her. I didn't realise because I made it into the lavatory in double-quick time, but apparently the whole court had emptied barring the legal team, who continued boldly on as though nothing had happened. The reports in the following day's papers read that I had run out in distress. I did, but that particular distress was eased simply by emptying my bladder. My mum, who also wanted to go to the loo, and Clare Dyer, the *Guardian* reporter I'd given my first interview to, were the only people who actually followed me into the cramped court toilets. Clare came to warn us that all the reporters were standing outside waiting to see me collapse or something equally dramatic. We shared the simple truth that I'd just needed a wee. She laughed and, by the time we went back outside, they'd obviously all realised and gone back into court. If it wasn't for Clare Dyer and Neil's later description of the mayhem I'd caused, I would have been completely unaware.

Fortunately, I didn't really miss anything. The judge had finishing reading out his judgement and Lord Lester was just getting on his feet. Sir Stephen Brown looked a bit confused. It was obvious that he had thought it was all over, but Lord Lester asked for leave to appeal. The judge told Lord Lester that this was an unnecessary question. He appeared to think that I had an automatic right to appeal, but Lord Lester replied that respectfully he did need to make the request and he could tell the court that the HFEA were about to oppose it.

The reasons the HFEA gave for this appeared rather strange. I couldn't really believe my ears when their barrister said they felt that the matter had been decided and that granting leave would only prolong my agony, cost me more money and would not be in my best interests. Fortunately, Sir Stephen Brown would hear none of it. He granted leave immediately with no hesitation. My relief and gratitude were overwhelming.

Next we asked to drop the anonymity order, which was dispensed with equally as quickly, and then we came to costs.

The HFEA's barrister stood on her feet to request their costs, but before she could open her mouth, Sir Stephen Brown interjected: 'I suppose you're about to tell me that, as you're a public body, you have to ask for your costs.'

'My Lord, that's right, but . . .'

'So, if I tell you that I'm not awarding them, that's the end of your problem.'

'My Lord, no. There's more to it than that. We have a finite budget and we feel . . .'

The judge abruptly told her that he thought she'd better sit down.

I'd lost, but I'd come out of the judgement with a victory I hadn't gone in with. Throughout my whole court ordeal I rarely saw my husband's face, felt his pain, anguish or elation. It was something I went through alone. But he always worried about money more than me and this one time I could almost feel the wind rush past my ears as he jumped up by my side and punched the air with his fist. *Good 'un, Di. You'll get there in the end.*

For now, I didn't have to pay the HFEA's costs and, best of all, I could appeal. Under the circumstances, 17 October turned out, quite simply, to be the best day I could have had – and it wasn't even over yet.

CHAPTER 10

A whirlwind of interviews

This time, all the reporters wanted me to leave the court by one of the rear entrances. Each bidder wanted to whisk me away in their own personal limousine, so they could wring out the exclusive before I spoke to everyone else. In the spirit of openness and equality, I wanted to follow my usual method of walking straight out the front. Everyone kept telling me of the hordes of photographers outside. They feared I might be crushed. Fortunately, a little ingenuity, planning and the essential help of the BBC's Joshua Rozenberg won the day for equal reporting opportunities.

There are some barriers in front of the High Court. The photographers are not meant to cross this line. The police are on hand to keep them in check, but when there is such a big crowd, the task is impossible. Even with the best of law-abiding intentions, the reporters closest to the barriers would be unintentionally pushed over the mark by those at the back. Joshua Rozenberg basically managed to cut a deal with everyone. I would come out the front and stand in relative safety on the steps, just behind the barriers. I would allow time for photographs to be taken and speak briefly to the reporters. Those with microphones could arrange their equipment inside the barriers. In return, no one would push forward and I could then go back inside the court building and leave by a side entrance.

The plan worked brilliantly. We made our way to the front

entrance, where a representative from the media met us and told us that everything was set up and ready. The idea of stepping out into the big wide world from the relative safety of the court was pretty daunting. There was obviously quite a crowd and we could hear them jostling and shouting instructions to one another. Still, we couldn't hang around too long because we knew they were waiting.

May as well get it over and done with. A few deep breaths and then we stepped forward with purpose. The bright sunlight and cool fresh wind came as quite a shock to the system. It is so dark in the High Court foyer. My pupils desperately tried to adjust and take in the sight before me. I was stunned by the sheer number of reporters. It was all rather bewildering and I felt terribly vulnerable. I imagine it's what a baby must feel like on leaving the warm, dark protection of its mother's womb to be thrust suddenly into the awaiting world.

I answered a few questions and expressed my deep disappointment at the decision. The reporters would have kept me there and had me hold a full conference on the court steps, if I'd let them, but I politely declined to go into further detail at that point and invited them to the press conference to be held later at the Waldorf Hotel. They seemed satisfied with that and we managed to leave quietly with no one hassling me or in pursuit.

We had a couple of hours in which to collect ourselves before the afternoon session. With nowhere else to go in the meantime, we headed straight for the Waldorf. I hadn't felt like eating for weeks. Now, I suddenly realised I was starving. Someone kindly volunteered to go and get some sandwiches.

It was quite bizarre, really, because we were there before all the reporters and sat in full view eating lunch while they poured in. No one bothered, photographed or hurried us. I don't really know what I expected, but with the bad reports I'd heard of the press, I was pleasantly surprised they let us eat in peace and respected the privacy of this time.

After lunch, I practised my calm breathing exercises and fidgeted nervously. No one reported it. Yet I knew any emotion I displayed on entering the press conference room would have been described. This seemed reasonable to me. If you draw some boundaries and tell people where they are, you should be able to step outside them and no longer be on show without having to hide yourself away. I was incredibly grateful for this consideration.

The only interruption to our lunch was the mobile phones. Calls from the media still trying to buy exclusive rights were interspersed with the occasional call regarding work. The classified sales rep from some trade magazine or other urgently needed to know if my client wished to take advantage of this month's amazing offer. It was hard to respond with my usual enthusiasm. One second I was turning down six-figure sums and the next I was dealing with a call which, if I was lucky, might make me a tenner. The financial considerations aside, it sort of put everything into perspective and made me question the validity and importance of life's mundane detail.

It was also at this point that I suddenly remembered that perhaps I ought to speak to my wedding photographer and ask him not to release exclusive photos. By the time I got through to him, he'd already heard the reports and realised he had the copyright on our wedding photos. According to my wishes, he sent selected photos out to a news syndicate, so everyone could have access to them from the following day. I hoped this might keep everyone sweet, whilst keeping the photos off the front pages the next day. As far as I was concerned, our wedding day was irrelevant to the news element of the story.

The plan for releasing the photos a day late was a bad one and in any case went awry when one of the photos was 'leaked' almost immediately. This caused a certain amount of confusion and panic, with everyone fighting for the one available photo from whatever source they could obtain it. With hindsight, I realise I should have released all the photos at once, with unhindered access. When I was told what was happening, I actually tried to revoke my earlier request. By this time, however, I couldn't contact the photographer.

With everyone now ready and waiting in the appointed room for the conference to commence, we took one last phone call. It was from a newspaper finally offering the one deal I'd previously stated I would consider: they would fund the appeal.

It came too late to warrant serious contemplation. If I'd run off without speaking to everyone at that point, can you imagine the mayhem it would have caused? If they'd later decided to come up with a contract that was not quite as they had verbally stated, I would already have turned everyone else against me and I'd be in no position to bargain. Call me cynical, but not only was it not worth the risk, to be honest, I'd been so impressed with the integrity of all the reporters so far that day that I felt pleased with the decision to work with them all. I was certainly not about to double-cross them at this point in the proceedings.

A few more steady breathing exercises and I began to work my way to the room we'd booked for the conference. Knowing that by opening your mouth you are about to say goodbye to several hundred thousand pounds which you desperately need is not easy.

Of course, I wasn't exchanging it for nothing. We were hoping to raise some money by launching the Stephen Blood Baby Appeal. I was swapping the certainty of a large amount of cash for the wing and prayer that God, the British public, some benevolent wealthy person or organisation, or a combination of all four, would somehow provide for my needs. Used in its broader sense, I was begging. I couldn't believe that the High Court's decision was just and I desperately wanted help to reverse its consequences. I was happy to accept that help in whatever form it might come and I was too distressed to care how pathetic I looked pleading for it. Money was such a small part of it; I also wanted support. I had been offered so much money for my story that I didn't particularly see giving it away for nothing and then welcoming donations as any kind of immoral gain of money. I was hurt when I later received hate mail from someone suggesting this. I just thought I was selling it directly to those who agreed with me enough to want to give something.

The press conference was incredibly hard work. From the moment I crossed the line into the room, the lights glared up and the cameras rolled. It was more intimidating than one can possibly imagine. Not because of any hostility, but the lights and flashes were so bright that I could not see those who were addressing me. It reminded me of those films where the interrogator shines a hot bright light into the subject's eyes. The fact that I believed there was no malice did not make the process any easier.

Paul Plant, Stephen's former work colleague, spoke first, opening the conference and launching the Stephen Blood Baby Appeal. Then I took the hotseat. Paul asked reporters to put their hands in the air and state where they were from before asking a question. This was helpful. If you can't see someone terribly well, at least a brief introduction helps give some kind of sketch of the person you are talking to.

The formal questions didn't last too long. We then broke up the conference, giving the reporters a brief amount of time to question me individually. The lights were turned off and the battery packs whirred to a halt. Everyone breathed out in unison. You could hear the tension being expelled. It wasn't just me who'd been on edge. It was as though everyone was relieved that they could now relax and question me without everyone else listening.

In reality, there were so many reporters wanting to see me that each one only got a few seconds. Envelopes and messages from various editors and producers were constantly being stuffed into my hand throughout the whole proceedings. *Will you do this programme, will you do that programme, can so and so have an interview?* I couldn't think, let alone work out the logistics of what was possible or desirable. In the end, I sort of thrust them all in the direction of Paul and Neil, who was also helping out at the conference, and left it to them to coordinate and decide what I would do. They did an admirable job of scheduling and the informal question session was finally brought to a halt by them telling me I had to leave to go to a TV studio for the evening news. We left, promising to return again tomorrow, when we had booked two small conference rooms: one for interviews and the other to use as a waiting room.

I was duly bundled into a taxi and off we went to Millbank studios. Fortunately, all the major stations, including Sky, work out of one set of studios, so I could make it live on all the channels virtually simultaneously. I was led from one room to the next. I felt a bit like a zombie on a production line. I guess it was the mental equivalent of being punch drunk.

Whenever someone judged I had a few seconds between interviews, I was wheeled into make-up, where someone did their best to make me look presentable. But 'What shade of lipstick do you normally wear?' seemed far too complicated and irrelevant a question for me at this point.

'Just do whatever you think,' came my somewhat vacant response.

This was my first experience of auto-cameras. I was put into my first room and told that in a few seconds this box would speak to me. I had to look at the lens above it, speak back and I'd be on TV. The idea of engaging in conversation with an inanimate object freaked me out somewhat, so I asked the girl who'd taken me to the room to stand at the side of the camera so I could 'speak' to her.

As a result, I probably looked cross-eyed, as well as shell shocked, but I have to say I really didn't care.

My opposition were being interviewed, too. As their Chairwoman, Ruth Deech spoke for the HFEA, but there were other organisations too. I remember contributions from Life (a pro-life charity) and The Society for the Protection of the Unborn Child. I usually caught the tail-end of their arguments on the run up to mine, so I generally started each session with a list of things buzzing around in my head that I needed to refute before we even started on what the interviewer wished to ask me.

Both Ruth Deech and Life appeared to think that attempting to secure my husband's reproductive future had stripped him of the opportunity for a dignified death. Life said that 'taking the sperm had violated the man's dignity and integrity'. Ruth Deech's comments were reported the following day in *The Times*, 'One shouldn't forget the husband in this case was totally unconscious and I think clinically dead when the sperm was taken from him . . . We must enable people to keep their dignity and their autonomy.' For my part, I simply pointed out that dying of meningitis could never have been dignified and that my husband and I became one the day we got married.

Overall, the lack of written consent from my late husband featured quite lightly in the list of objections to the treatment I desired. Those who opposed me, including Ruth Deech, also cited more general concerns about posthumous conception. Many of them felt it was wrong to deliberately bring a child into the world without a father, as well as to create a living memorial to a deceased loved one in the form of a child. Ruth Deech later raised the question in an interview for the *New Statesman*: 'As thousands of young people die every year, would taking sperm become the natural reaction to a sudden death?' They appeared to think that I wanted my late husband's offspring because he had died. I thought this was ridiculous and pointed out that I still wanted his baby *in spite* of the fact that he had died, not because of it. We were trying for a baby before his death. I wanted that child now for the same reasons as I did before the tragic loss of my husband.

I became particularly frustrated when nearly everyone began by expressing sympathy and then demonstrating none whatsoever. They seemed to think that it was our fault that my husband and I hadn't had children before he died – as though leaving a small child grieving for a father they had briefly known was somehow a better option. We should have had children sooner, after all we had had a twelve-year relationship prior to Stephen's death. I pointed out that the first eight years or so were before we were married, then immediately after our wedding I had found myself out of work, but that we were trying for a child at the time of his death.

I was just 16 when I met Steph. It seemed that a teenage unmarried girl having a baby was preferable to the prospect of a widow becoming a mother. Of course I would do things differently if we had our time again, but I had thought I had followed the sensible path dictated by society. Despite falling in love at a young age, I'd waited until the week after my 25th birthday before marrying (the average age for a woman to marry in 1991 was 24). I had built a career and some financial stability and then begun trying for a family at 28, which was again pretty average. I hadn't done anything out of the ordinary. But for the grace of God, anyone could have found themselves in my position. The implication that I had somehow brought this tragedy on myself really hurt.

The tears pricked at the back of my eyes, but I tried to remain collected and coherent. I made the points I wanted to make and, miraculously, I managed not to miss any of my allocated slots. By the time I'd got to the end, I even felt happier about those stupid auto-cameras. I'd graduated from having to have someone stand at the side, but now I'd developed a tendency to speak at the box rather than the camera. As this was usually positioned below the lens, I probably looked as if I had my eyes closed. I was operating on pure adrenalin. The whole thing has merged into a huge blurred buzz in the recess of my memory. It was OK until I stopped.

Newsnight was my last port of call. For this one, we had to go in a taxi to a different studio. It was a reasonably lengthy journey, but I haven't a clue where we went. Being October and fairly late at night, it was dark, but even if it had been broad daylight, I might as well have been blindfolded. I was still in a daze. Jeremy Paxman, the interviewer, met me at the door, which was kind of him. I'm just sorry I didn't show my appreciation.

The pace slowed down somewhat, which was a bit of a problem for me. I'd been doing non-stop live interviews for a good few hours. I'd been constantly bombarded with questions. Jeremy Paxman was too nice and tried his best to put me at ease. It threw me completely, especially as he has such a reputation for being a harsh interviewer.

Unlike the others, this interview wasn't quite live, although it was recorded in one go, almost as if it were. I'm told I came across really well. I don't know. Despite just being back at the hotel in time for it to be transmitted, I didn't watch it, which I now regret. The people from the studio were even kind enough to ring me in my hotel room right before it was broadcast, but I just couldn't face it. I'd had enough. On leaving the *Newsnight* studios, I'd run into my mum's arms, cried my eyes out and told everyone it had gone really badly.

One particular reason for regretting not watching the *Newsnight* interview was the practical consideration of sorting out the mayhem that it caused the following day. Apparently, Ruth Deech had denied that they had offered not to apply for costs to be awarded against me if I didn't appeal. Basically, it looked as if it was her word against mine – except it wasn't really because, apart from my full legal team, there had been five of us in the room when the offer was made to me.

Clare Dyer, from *The Guardian*, decided to investigate and my parents and Stephen's friends who had been present confirmed the accuracy of my testimony. The following morning, *The Guardian* reported that the HFEA had later admitted that the offer had been made, but said that Ruth Deech had not been aware of it. This was one report that I did read. The whole thing had created such a stir and got both myself and my lawyers into quite a lot of bother, which seemed ridiculous really. All they did was communicate the proposal to me and all I did was tell the truth.

The problem, apparently, was that the offer had been made 'without prejudice', meaning that my lawyers were bound by their professional code not to discuss it with anyone (although quite how they were supposed to ask me to consider it without telling me what it was, I really don't know). It seemed that everyone was offended and rather annoyed that I had raised the issue in public. I still found it distasteful that the offer had been made in the first place and now I was even more upset at being made to look like a liar on TV, but this didn't seem to count. I didn't see why everyone should be left with the impression that I was untruthful. The offer was made, but it was denied on peak-time national TV and the denial only later retracted in a few small column inches in a daily newspaper. The report contained in *The Guardian* would have reached only a very small audience compared to *Newsnight*.

Apart from seeing Clare Dyer, the day after judgement was taken up with a constant stream of interviews with all and sundry. I think there were representatives from every British newspaper, as well as TV and foreign reporters. Most people got around a half-hour slot, but I did have one or two false starts. There were many aspects of my and my late husband's life which I saw as private and I didn't want to discuss. When reporters, perhaps unwittingly, encroached on these areas, I became upset because I didn't know how to politely draw the line. I thought that the finer details of our honeymoon were completely irrelevant to the situation now in question and I particularly remember one female reporter asking about our respective childhoods. I stumbled on my words. I started the sentence, but then it trailed into thin air. My dad got really angry with the woman, which I suppose was a bit unfair. The question had seemed innocent enough to her. I kept having to ask for a break to give me time to think exactly how much I wished to disclose.

As consideration for my time and story, we requested donations to the Stephen Blood Baby Appeal and we asked newspapers to print the details along with their article. Friends from an advertising agency had managed to produce our Appeal posters rather speedily. We stuck them up on the walls and asked the photographers to record them for artwork. Thankfully, most newspapers carried the information we desired, although many promises of cash donations from the publishers themselves never actually materialised.

Apart from the potential danger of allowing my privacy to be invaded and feeling somewhat uptight and on edge, I suppose I have had worse days. My flagging will was refuelled by the news that the Stephen Blood Baby Appeal phonelines had been jammed all day by people trying to call in. I even heard we had a single pledge from one company of £1,000, but no one could supply me with a running total. At the end of the day, when everyone had gone home, the best estimate turned out to be only just under the £3,000 mark. Many of the calls had been from media people or those just wanting more information. The rooms for the interviews had cost around £800 each and, in addition, I'd been landed with a hotel phone bill as a result of photographers using modems to transmit their pictures. They told me they had been using 0800 Freefone numbers, but apparently hotels still charge for these. We learnt from this one. At all press conferences in the future, we disconnected the phones.

We were lucky if we'd broken even. I could have cried my heart out. It had been such incredibly hard work. Having said that, at least the interviews gave my perspective on the story. The HFEA had been publicising their point of view. It would have been unbalanced without mine. I was also touched by some of the stories relayed to me from those who had pledged money. One couple donated the remainder of a fund set up to help their young daughter fight a life-threatening medical condition. Sadly, she had died. The money couldn't bring her back, so they wanted it to help someone else to have the opportunity to have the child they desperately wanted. I was very grateful.

At around teatime, I called it a day and decided not to do any more interviews. I was still being asked to appear on various TV shows, but I really couldn't have taken any more. Paul Plant, on the other hand, was still going strong and he agreed to travel up to Nottingham to appear on a TV discussion programme. My sister-in-law, Sue, and her husband also made their TV debut on this one. I had always thought that Sue was a fairly quiet, unassuming person. Apparently not. She got rather riled at what my opponents were saying, particularly when they started suggesting that my child would be an extra mouth for the state to feed. Sue pointed out that I worked and had always planned to continue working from home when I had a child. She managed to put across all our points quite forcefully and I was quite touched that she felt able to defend me so strongly.

I have to say, though, this programme rather put the whole media frenzy into perspective. One man, who was arguing vehemently against me, later privately admitted to Paul that he was doing so purely because he had been hired by the programme researchers to fulfil that role. He actually agreed with me, but, without controversy, there is no programme. What a farce.

Once you realise the way topical discussion shows work, you can never quite look at them in the same light again. Not that I ever really looked at them at all before I ended up being asked to appear on half of them. When you're not tied up in the middle of it all, it's actually quite amusing. You see the same faces over and over again in the audience of different chat shows. They join in the discussion and argue passionately. One week their background means they are uniquely qualified to offer a particular insight on one subject, next week it's something else. You begin to question why these people feel so strongly about so many different issues, and even though it's more obvious why the programme researchers constantly recruit the same people, it is still upsetting when you are involved. To me, it was all so terribly important. To others, well I guess it was just a job or, even worse, another excuse for self-promotion.

Still, whatever criticisms I may wish to make of the system, it appeared to work. People watched the programmes and despite, or perhaps because of, the HFEA and their supporters' stony opposition, people heard my plea. I begged politicians to help me and seconds later I would see some member of the House of Commons saying that, if they won the ballot, they would introduce a Private Member's Bill. Labour MP for Eccles Joan Lestor wanted to put forward a Bill to give more discretion in cases like mine, and Lord Winston decided to start action in the Lords, with the assistance of Baroness Warnock. I begged the public to write to anyone of influence. I didn't know until later, but write they did – in their hundreds. It is rather humbling to know that I am indebted to so many.

I also begged the HFEA to reconsider its stance. We had already asked this officially through my solicitors immediately before going to court, but they had refused to look at the evidence. I hoped the members were watching. It was the only way I could get to speak to them.

Finally, after two days of solid interviews, we escaped London to head back home. On the way back, I received a call on my mobile from the *Daily Express*. They had gained inside information that the Government would not block a Private Member's Bill and the accuracy of this had been confirmed. 'Whitehall sources said that Health Secretary Stephen Dorrell would not stand in the way of moves to change the law', and it was reported that 'Health Minister John Horam, who is responsible for medical ethics, took a close interest in the case and sent Government lawyers to monitor progress'. I was cautiously happy and tremendously grateful to them for bringing me this news, but the front-page headline in the following morning's paper which began: 'Exclusive: Widow can have baby' was far from the truth. To be honest, not being au fait with the finer points of politics, I wasn't really sure of the implications of all they had said, but the *Express* told me it meant the law could be changed really quickly. I now know that the speed of a Private Member's Bill is a matter of comparison only. Without Government backing, it can still take many, many years.

The effect of the overly optimistic *Express* headline, however, soon became obvious. When I got home, everyone started congratulating me, thinking I'd won. Money going in to the Stephen Blood Baby Appeal immediately dried up. People thought I no longer needed it and much of the money that was initially pledged was never actually transferred.

The repercussions of this headline were so great that I, cynical as ever, even thought it might have been a deliberate ploy by the Government to stop everyone talking about the subject. Artificial human reproduction is a bit of a hot potato at the best of times, but with a general election looming it would be a particularly unwelcome topic. The original passage of the Human Fertilisation and Embryology Act was delayed because of the desire not to discuss the controversial issue before a general election. This is not my opinion. It's historical fact, recorded in the relevant Hansard Debates on several occasions.

Once it had started, the tidal wave of inaccurate opinion from those who thought I had won was particularly difficult to stem. I was back in Nottinghamshire and had agreed to an interview with Sue Lawley for the Current Affairs programme *Here and Now* on Sunday, but I was too exhausted to do anything else.

The reporters, however, had other ideas. They wouldn't let me rest.

CHAPTER 11

Taking our plight
to the House of Commons

I returned home once again to find a huge pile of letters on my doormat. Most carried very little information by way of address, but the Royal Mail somehow still managed to find me. Most letters offered sympathy and outrage at the court's decision. It made a huge difference to me, as I didn't feel so alone. In the end, for the hundreds of supportive letters I received from all over the world, including France, Zambia, New Zealand, Canada and the USA, I received a total of six from people who were opposed to what I was trying to do. Although the people who sent these obviously did not sign their names, it was clear that three of these abusive letters were from the same woman.

After reading all the letters, I stuffed them hurriedly into drawers in the hope that I might one day have the time and space to file them somewhere more sensible. The reporters were still chasing me for comments on the *Express* story about changing the law. It was difficult, as at the same time I was trying to mentally prepare for the interview with Sue Lawley for *Here and Now*. My home was like Bedlam. It's only a two-bedroom bungalow. Far too small to house chaos.

Sunday morning arrived, along with a film crew, both my own and Stephen's parents, both Stephen's sisters and their families. Then Sue Lawley arrived. And the phone still wouldn't stop ringing. In the end, the film crew pulled it out of the socket, accidentally wiping all the messages on the answerphone at the same time. I don't like people messing with my belongings at the best of times, but I found losing my messages, which I hadn't had the chance to listen to, really upsetting. Little things can take on gigantic proportions when you're feeling down in the first place.

Sue Lawley was lovely, even though I was a total wreck by the time she arrived. She even diplomatically suggested that perhaps we should escape into my bedroom so I could put some make-up on. She said that, although she appreciated that make-up wasn't exactly top of my agenda at that moment in time, ultimately I would care. I supposed she was right, so I hurriedly applied some.

The interview was OK but difficult because Sue Lawley is a good interviewer. She asks the same question over and over again, using slightly different words, until she either gets the answer she wants or is satisfied that the one you're giving really must be the truth, the whole truth and nothing but the truth. It was tiring and I was glad when it was over. What I was not so happy about was that Sue's researcher and driver accidentally backed into my front wall when they were leaving, knocking off one of the slabs on the way out of the drive. The girl apologised profusely and offered to pay for the wall to be fixed. It really was no big deal. It just needed a bit of cement to stick the slab back on, but at the time it was just something else I could have done without. I told her it didn't matter, but I had to work quite hard to remind myself that it really didn't.

We plugged the phone back in. It was still ringing. Also, one or two reporters began turning up at my door. We decided I was going to have to say something, so we called The Innings, a local pub, arranged to borrow a room and dispatched the reporters off to wait for me, promising that I would give a press conference shortly.

Hastily, we scribbled down something that I could say and called my solicitor to check it out. It wasn't anything very earth-shattering. Basically, just that I was pleased the Government wouldn't block a Bill, but the fight wasn't over yet and I'd be pursuing my action through the courts. I didn't really know what else I could say. The reporters, however, wanted to know every last little detail. I turned up at the conference, read the piece I had prepared and then they started to ask questions. I opened my mouth to respond to the first one, but the words didn't come out.

I was just too exhausted to think, let alone speak any more. Paul, from the Stephen Blood Baby Appeal, who was there with me, explained that I was tired from doing a previously arranged interview in the morning and that I therefore wouldn't be answering questions. This really annoyed everyone. Apparently, if I wasn't going to answer questions, I should have called it a press statement and not a press conference. Not only did I not know this, I also hadn't known until I'd got there that I was basically just too shattered to take any more. Everyone left in a bad humour and it's not really a good idea to upset reporters when you need them.

The next morning I was woken by the telephone at some ridiculously early hour. It was one of the press syndicates. Apparently, there had been a report in *The Guardian* about a woman who had been refused the opportunity to take a sample of her dying husband's sperm. She and her husband had been having problems conceiving naturally and had visited a fertility clinic. They were due to go ahead with the treatment but hadn't yet signed the forms when her husband had been killed in a tragic car accident. She had been refused the chance to take his sperm because we were still waiting for the outcome of my court case. I felt awful, as though it was all my fault. If it hadn't been for my case, they would have taken her husband's sperm. I didn't comment, saying that I wanted a chance to read the article.

There was more to come. A woman from Chesterfield phoned me and begged me to hear her out before I hung up. Her husband had died of a brain haemorrhage five months after I'd lost my husband. He'd died in the Hallamshire, the same hospital as Stephen. She too had asked if they could take some sperm. She had been refused. Someone had apparently even suggested that, as an alternative, she should try having sex with her husband as he lay dying on the ward. As you can imagine, she'd felt particularly aggrieved. She was 38 and worked with children. It was probably her last chance to have a child of her own. If I hadn't got there first, they'd have taken her husband's sperm, as they had done Steph's. At least I still had a chance. She wasn't at all bitter towards me, however, and she wished me luck.

I began to crumble with the burden of everyone else's loss. By now the rest of the world had got up and had also read the *Guardian* article. All the newspapers were ringing for my comments. After the first couple of callers, who I promised to get back to when I'd seen the article, I knew what the calls were about, so I didn't answer the phone. It was such a horrible din. I sat there clutching a cushion, crying my eyes out, rocking gently back and forth, like a toddler seeking comfort. But the phone wouldn't stop ringing. The second it stopped, it started again. What could I say? I'm so sorry I was lucky enough to be first? I wasn't. It was just such a shame we all couldn't have had our husbands' sperm stored. If it had been someone else who had managed to get the sperm and not me, I wondered if they'd have had the resolve to take it to court. It wasn't my fault, but I found it very hard to deal with how events in my life had affected these other unfortunate women.

Between rings, I managed to grab the phone long enough to call my parents, blurt my problems down the phone to them and ask them if they could buy a copy of *The Guardian* and bring it up. This they did. They suggested pulling the phone out of the socket again, but, having just reprogrammed the stupid thing, I felt rather reluctant to do this. I was determined not to let the situation get the better of me. To have unplugged my phone would have meant I was allowing the journalists to rule my life. I'd bought the phone. I'd paid for the line rental. Why, then, should I voluntarily disconnect it?

The only solution seemed to be to answer the questions and get it over and done with, so we organised another press conference down at the pub. This time we were careful not to confuse a press conference with a statement. I was feeling pretty emotional anyway, so that afternoon I probably gave away more about myself than I did at any other conference throughout the whole court proceedings. I was frightened of upsetting everyone again and I badly wanted the journalists' support to help change the law, not only for myself now but for other women too.

My local MP Joe Ashton finally decided to join in the media frenzy. He added his support to the campaign and managed to get a debate in the House of Commons scheduled for 30 October, a week on Wednesday. At the end of the debate, the Parliamentary Under-Secretary of State for Health, John Horam, would give a response, so it might even prompt some action. We quickly had to brief Mr Ashton and I had to have a bit of a crash induction into parliamentary lobbying and the mechanics of government.

There is not exactly a lot you can do in a little over a week, but we did what we could. The *Here and Now* programme, which had originally been scheduled to go out the Wednesday after judgement, was put back a week to maximise publicity, both for the programme and the campaign to change the law. It would now go out on the same day as the debate and would be trailered from the weekend before. We also arranged a press conference for after the debate. The landlord of one of the pubs on Fleet Street kindly offered to lend us a room for the venue.

The Stephen Blood Baby Appeal wrote to all the members of the Commons, informing them of the debate, outlining a few salient points and asking them to attend. Unfortunately, due to the limited amount of time and the fact that most of the MPs are not permanently in the Commons to read their mail, most of them didn't get our letter until after the debate had taken place.

In the meantime, the offers to buy my story or for me to appear on various programmes around the world still kept flooding in. I was asked to fly out to America to go on the *Oprah Winfrey Show,* but it was the same day as the Commons debate, so I refused, promising to do it later. I was asked to appear on *Heart of the Matter,* with Joan Bakewell; I said I'd think about it. Every time I refused to do a programme, I was desperately afraid that the debate would still take place without my opinion being represented and the programme makers would only report the opposing view because they had taken umbrage at my refusal to help them. It was a very delicate line to tread and I hated the indecision and fear that it created.

The day of the Commons debate was soon upon us. We had been given tickets to attend and my father and I were travelling down to London on the train. My mum decided to avoid the inevitable media frenzy and stayed at home to watch the debate on TV.

Here and Now were still gathering material for their programme that night, so they met us on the train at Peterborough and filmed us going down. The rest of the media pack were already waiting for me outside the Commons and my solicitor, Richard Stein, was meeting us at King's Cross.

He had the most amazing news for me. The previous evening, the HFEA's solicitors had faxed my solicitor's office to inform us that the HFEA had decided to reconsider their stance on export. They gave us a deadline for a couple of weeks' time, asking me to submit any evidence I wished them to consider by that date. I could hardly believe it. The members of the HFEA must have heard my pleas on television asking them to reconsider. Before the court case they'd refused, but now they'd obviously decided to take on board the individual circumstances of my case. I was surprised and overjoyed.

My father and I discussed the new development briefly with my solicitor, but it was a bit difficult because the *Here and Now* film crew were with us, so we were trying to talk without being overheard. Our secret didn't last very long. No sooner had we left King's Cross and scrambled into a taxi than the mobiles started ringing: both ours and the film crew's. The HFEA had just put it out on the wires that they were going to reconsider the export question and that John Horam was to announce it at the end of the Commons debate. Everyone wanted to know my opinion. I was a bit flummoxed because we hadn't had time to think it through thoroughly. We tried to look for a downside, but it seemed to be a genuine response both to my obvious distress and to the concern that the public had shown over my plight. In the light of the evidence, everyone had said the HFEA should reconsider and now they'd agreed. What was there to be cynical about? It looked like I was home and dry.

This new twist in the tale totally defused the effect of the Commons debate. What was there left to debate, when someone had effectively already said, 'Hang on, give us a bit more time and we'll look at it again?' The Government could hardly intervene when the HFEA had agreed to revisit the issue themselves. Perhaps the HFEA and the Government were already in cahoots and this was the line they'd agreed to take. After all, John Horam had obviously known about it way before anyone else, as he had had to prepare his speech. Whatever the case, I didn't really care so long as this time the HFEA came up with the right answer.

We met Joe Ashton inside Westminster. He introduced me to Tessa Jowell, another Labour MP who was going to speak on my behalf. Lord Winston was also there. He had come to listen to the debate. I also met up with a former work colleague of mine, Jonathan, who'd been a guest at my wedding. He now worked in London and did the occasional bit of parliamentary lobbying, so he'd come along to lend support and, if he could, give a bit of advice as to the implications of what was being said. This was useful because I knew I was going to have to discuss my opinion about it all when it was over. We all exchanged greetings and then quickly made our way to our various posts for the debate. Lord Winston, Jonathan, my dad and I were upstairs, watching from the gallery.

Joe Ashton opened the proceedings. The next MP to speak, Dame Jill Knight (Birmingham Edgbaston) really annoyed and upset me. Everyone is entitled to their opinion, but what particularly irritated me was that this woman claimed to have sympathy and understand exactly how I felt because she'd lost her husband too. She was a middle-aged matriarch-type figure, who sounded like she was chastising a wayward child. She was not at all on my wavelength and certainly wasn't young enough to even begin to understand how it might feel to be widowed at 28 in 1995. She thought that the potential child 'had the right to expect the law to protect them' as they were so 'utterly vulnerable' and had 'no say in whether they are to be born'. She stated that my child would have to 'take on board the fact that he was born as the child of a dead man, and not until many months after his father's death'. This, she insisted, 'would be enough to cause nightmares in that child'. She spoke with such authority that she seemed to think that everyone would naturally agree with her. I couldn't make my mind up whether she sounded like a schoolteacher preaching to her class or an overgrown school child having a strop.

She obviously irritated her colleague too. Dame Elaine Kellett-Bowman, MP for Lancaster, stood up just behind her, interjecting that she normally agreed with her honourable friend, but, on this occasion, she couldn't help but strongly disagree. 'He will not have nightmares.'

'A sensitive child might well have nightmares at the certain knowledge that he was born from a dead man. That frightens me,' was the response from Dame Jill Knight.

The sharp exchange seemed ill-researched and unnecessary. Milo Casali, the child of the first woman to conceive posthumously in Britain, was born in 1977. Both he and his mother, Kim, had communicated their support for me in the *Daily Mail*. Cancer robbed Milo Casali of his father, but, as Kim Casali put it, 'at least he got his chance at life' and it would be 'a terrible thought' if he had not.

Although Kim believed that posthumous conception was only something she would recommend to a woman who already had children, on the grounds that a childless woman could have a family from a new relationship, Milo disagreed. 'There shouldn't be any opposition, whatever the wife's situation. If a woman loses her husband, it should be her decision alone. I don't find it immoral or unethical for a woman to use her dead husband's sperm to have the family they expected to have if he had lived, even if they don't already have children.'

Why hadn't anyone thought to ask him if he'd had nightmares? I'm sure he would have said if the circumstances of his birth had left him mentally scarred. Yet he was reported to be 'a sensitive and thoughtful young man with a great future'. To have such an ill-informed debate about the psychological effects of posthumous conception almost 20 years after Milo's birth seemed to deny his very existence.

The next couple of speakers seemed to go off at a bit of a tangent, managing to turn the debate into an anti-abortion issue, discussing the unnecessary destruction of embryos. I had already discovered that pro-life groups were also very strongly opposed to posthumous conception. This suprised me at first, until I discovered that they have incredibly loud voices on a number of different issues. In fact, almost anything that can relate back to abortion. I would have thought they'd have been for life, not against it. My husband didn't agree with abortion and, whilst I would never condemn anyone who had an abortion because of their particular circumstances, I wouldn't exactly view it as a method of contraception either. It amazed me that on one issue we could almost agree (although definitely not with their ferocity of approach) and yet on another we were poles apart. I really could not understand the arguments put against me.

I am obviously biased in my opinion and perhaps I am overly critical of those who disagree with my point of view. I do not mean to sound bitter. It is, in part, a defence mechanism against the pain it caused at the time. The whole experience of laying my emotions open to scrutiny was like living with a knife permanently protruding from my stomach. Every time someone said, 'I have every sympathy, BUT,' the knife turned, grinding mercilessly at the sinew. I could taste the blood. I sometimes wished they would shut up just long enough for me to catch my breath.

That experience over, Tessa Jowell wound up the proceedings with an uplifting speech and then John Horam basically announced that it had all been pretty irrelevant, as the HFEA were going to reconsider their decision anyway. End of debate – end of story. I only wish.

The reporters were waiting for us outside the House of Commons. We gave a few quick comments and then got whisked away by *Here and Now* for a few more questions to finish their programme. It was quite nice to relax for a while as they set up their cameras. They got us some sandwiches and left us in peace to eat our lunch and discuss the morning's events amongst ourselves.

Next on the agenda was the press conference back at the pub on Fleet Street. When we'd organised it, we hadn't envisaged there being quite so much interest, so we'd not paid too much attention to the size of the room. It wasn't that small, but, all the same, it was crammed full. We arrived slightly late, as we had been delayed longer than expected with the *Here and Now* crew. Consequently, everyone was already set up and waiting, and there were several people with mobiles posted outside watching for my arrival. The police were also outside the pub. I wondered what on earth was going on and half considered turning back and heading in the opposite direction, but apparently the police had just thought they better be on hand because of the sheer number of people at the venue. Either that or they just wanted to get in on the act.

We made our way upstairs to the waiting throng. The vast interest had been created because of the news that the HFEA were to reconsider their position. The reporters seemed as euphoric as I was. They even got as far as starting to ask questions like, 'What was I going to call the child?' or 'Would I like twins?'

The thought of a child still seemed like a distant dream, as there were the medical hurdles still to overcome, but all the same I allowed myself a flicker of a smile.

Only one reporter thought to ask, 'What if all is not as it seems? Have you thought they could just be trying to bolster their case for the appeal?' Of course, that thought had occurred to me, but I'd dismissed it as being unduly cynical. It was my father who answered the question. 'If they would play around with my daughter's emotions in that manner, well, it just beggars belief.' The reporter nodded in agreement and the moment's solemnity passed.

When the conference was over, we went downstairs to thank the landlord for the use of the room and grab a very welcome drink. Many of the journalists hung around too, penning their articles over a glass of beer. They didn't hassle us. They just got on with their work, although one did ask if I'd mind confirming my age, as he wasn't sure if he'd got it right. If I hadn't been looking at him at the time, I don't think he'd have bothered to ask. It was strange to see the journalists relaxed. In a conference situation they always seemed almost as uptight as me. The journalist smiled, 'Don't tell anyone I told you, but, off the record, the word on the street is that many members of the HFEA are with you. We think you're gonna get what you want.'

I smiled back, but he wasn't looking for a reaction. We both knew he couldn't report it.

We headed back to King's Cross, grabbing a copy of the *Evening Standard* on the way. I'd made the front page. It was strange to think my photo was in print before I'd even left the pub. It was nice to see a happy story for a change.

Now all that remained was to get back home and hope that the *Here and Now* programme went all right that evening. Mum was going to record it, as we wouldn't be back in time.

We took our seats and watched in amusement as the passengers streamed on, clutching their newspapers and doing a double-take when they realised the person on the front page was sitting on the train. Some of them offered their congratulations. Everyone thought I'd won again. The difference was that, this time, so did I.

During the journey, I had a rather pleasant feeling of tiredness, mixed with contentment. I couldn't remember the last time I'd felt so good. I interlocked my fingers and stretched my arms out in front of me, feeling, I imagine, rather like a cat stretching out on the hearth for the first time after being shut out in the cold. I thought that the hard work was over. It had paid off and I would soon be allowed to get on with the rest of my life and try for the child Steph and I had wanted so much.

Once we'd left behind the tunnels just after King's Cross, I called my mum from my mobile to give her the lowdown on the day's events. Not that she wouldn't already know from the TV. It was useless trying to speak to her, however, because clips from mine and Stephen's wedding video had just been on *Here and Now* and she was in tears. Steph and I had been dancing to 'Endless Love'.

She told me the programme and the interviews with myself and my parents-in-law had come over very well. 'It was good.'

'I had a good day too, Mum. I'll tell you about it when we get home.'

CHAPTER 12

The HFEA reconsider

Now that the HFEA had agreed to reconsider their decision on export, from the beginning of November 1996 it seemed wrong to continue doing interviews. Of course the money coming into the Appeal fund had dried up again, but it didn't really matter, as I genuinely didn't think I was going to need it. *Heart of the Matter* were still waiting for me to get back to them about doing their programme for the BBC. The proposed format was a ten-minute film broadcasting my point of view and then a two-part discussion, the first half with me taking part in the debate and then the second half without me. It seemed a reasonable opportunity to promote my opinion on a well-respected programme, but I called to explain that, with my fate hanging in the balance, as it currently was, I didn't feel able to oblige.

I was therefore absolutely horrified when they then rang to tell me they were going to go ahead with the programme anyway and make it from the opposing perspective. It was like my worst nightmare come true. Robert Snowdon, a former member of the HFEA who strongly opposed my point of view, had agreed to make a ten-minute film highlighting his disapproval of posthumous birth. He was going to introduce, as an example, a young man whose girlfriend had tragically died whilst pregnant. His wish to turn off her life-support machine had been overruled, as the baby was still alive, and both the doctors and the girl's parents wanted the machine left on long enough for the baby to be delivered. They would then widen the debate to discuss posthumous conception and cases such as mine. If such a programme was to be made, I at least wanted to defend myself and make sure the facts were correctly portrayed, but, at the time, I just felt I couldn't. It was so awkward and it really tore me apart, but I could hardly expect others not to broadcast their opinions for my convenience.

Most people couldn't understand why I was so upset. 'Well, you don't have to watch it' was a common comment.

I couldn't understand why anyone would expect me not to be deeply aggrieved. To me, it didn't seem fair that they would be effectively talking about me behind my back, but in front of several thousand TV viewers.

On 13 November, we submitted our arguments for the HFEA meeting. Once again I offered to meet them, but in anticipation that they would refuse I also wrote a personal letter to HFEA members imploring them to remember that 'I am a real human being who is already placed in the position I am in, at this point of time', and asking them 'to promote rather than thwart my husband's wishes'.

We tried to get an idea from the HFEA about when they would be making their decision or at least a date for when they would be meeting to discuss the subject. My solicitors wrote to them on several occasions. We received no reply. Fortunately, the Court of Appeal date had now been set for early January, less than a couple of months away. If it hadn't been for the fact that I knew they had to respond before then, the open-endedness of the whole procedure would have driven me mad.

Finally, at 5 p.m. on 20 November, my solicitors suddenly received a fax with a partial response. It still gave no date for the HFEA's meeting but said they would let me know their decision by Christmas. Not exactly a great improvement on January, but I was satisfied that I at least had some idea of their timeframe.

What I was not so happy about was another letter that accompanied the fax. It was a letter from Dr J. Stuart Horner, Chairman of the Medical Ethics Committee for the BMA (British Medical Association), to the HFEA, stating his opinions based on what he had read in the newspapers. The letter was dated 19 November. It was both damning and highly prejudicial. It urged the members of the HFEA to maintain their current stance and not allow me to export my husband's sperm. My solicitors and I were informed that the letter would be shown to members of the

HFEA and we were given until noon the following day to reply. They didn't give a reason for the short deadline, but I assumed it was because the original deadline when they had planned to have their arguments submitted by had already passed. They'd had all our other arguments on time but now needed to check if we specifically wished to respond to the new letter. It was like being handed a time bomb and being forced to hold it. *You have until noon tomorrow to defuse this. Fail, and it will explode.*

Factually, it was easy enough to attack his letter, as it was based on hearsay, without consideration of the actual court evidence itself. However, finding the right words and making sure you haven't missed anything when you have so much at stake is a pretty tough call. My legal team, myself and my family spent most of the evening on the phone. My parents and I then sat up all night working on a draft response to fax back to my solicitors the following morning. By 9 a.m., I was exhausted. Emotionally and physically, I think I'd pushed myself just about to the limit. I felt as though I needed to go to sleep for about a fortnight to catch up on the one night I'd missed.

Apart from the ridiculous deadline for a response, one of the most annoying things I found about the letter was that it was a single opinion based on newspaper reports. Looking at the contents of my own mailbag, I knew that the HFEA must have had tons of letters from all sorts of different people stating their views based on the same criteria as the letter at issue. Why should this one be singled out to be presented to the HFEA members whilst all the others were to be ignored?

I decided that if one letter was to be presented, they all should. My solicitors weren't too convinced about this one, as I obviously didn't know what the other letters said. They could all have been as damning as the one I was trying to defend, but I was adamant, no matter what they thought. The letters were written to the HFEA, so why shouldn't the members see all of them?

Consequently, the instructions were issued to the HFEA's solicitors that I wished all the letters that had been sent to them regarding my case to be presented along with the one from Dr Stuart Horner. This caused a certain amount of mayhem, because there were rather more of them than even I had anticipated and the HFEA's solicitors said that all the names and addresses would have to be removed from them first. I didn't really mind this, but it still seems a little peculiar to me that it was OK to leave the name and address on the letter from Dr Stuart Horner of the BMA, but all others had to be removed. Whoever the people were, they had written to the HFEA and chosen to include their names and addresses. I wasn't asking for them to be published in a newspaper, I merely asked that they be viewed by the very people they were addressed to: the members of the HFEA. For all I know, in their midst might have been a letter from someone who was very highly qualified, whose letter deserved more weight than anonymity afforded. Anyway, names and addresses were removed and I assume they were presented as I had requested. Copies were faxed to my solicitors for our files. Apart from the sheer quantity, I was also very pleasantly surprised that so many had written in my support.

Work continued throughout the morning on my reply to the BMA letter. I had had to go into the office because I had other things to do as well and I'd had no warning that I would need to take time out to deal with this important development on my court case. It was awkward trying to concentrate, but I thought that I would perhaps be able to get on better in the afternoon, when the HFEA's deadline had passed.

The morning was complicated further by a phone call from ITN, who were pretty insistent that they should be allowed to come up and sit with me. They had been told that the HFEA were having their meeting that afternoon and that there would be a press conference afterwards. They wanted to be with me when I was told the decision.

Considering that I had only just been told the evening before that the decision would be given by Christmas and we were still feverishly working away on evidence to be presented at a meeting for which we had no date, I, not surprisingly, thought that ITN had been misinformed. I told them so, but they still wanted to come up. Apparently, their information had come from the HFEA, although they admitted that it was because they knew someone and had the benefit of an inside source. I didn't have the energy to argue, so I told them they could come and waste their time if they wished, as long as they sat quietly in the office and didn't disturb me while I got on with my work.

The camera crew arrived just as I was faxing over the final response to the BMA letter. They clattered in with lights, cameras and trailing electrical cables.

'I hope you're not going to turn those things on. I'm trying to get on with some work.'

They promised not to film unless something happened and not without my prior permission, but they explained that they didn't wish to leave such expensive equipment outside in their vehicle.

It seemed that peace was determined to elude me that day. We ushered them into a rapidly vacated office, sat them down, gave them a drink and then tried to ignore their presence. It wasn't easy. What if they were right? What if the HFEA really were going to give a decision today? I dismissed the thought as nonsense, but as the day wore on the heat began to build. Other journalists began to call, confirming ITN's story. They told me that the HFEA had called a press conference for that evening. I immediately rang my solicitor, but he was out on other business. Relatives also began to call. ITN were broadcasting that a decision was to be announced later. Of course, my in-laws wanted to know why I hadn't told them. It seemed a little far-fetched when I had to explain that I didn't know.

About 4 p.m., I finally gave up trying to work altogether. ITN wanted to set up their cameras and I was becoming increasingly distraught. My solicitor still hadn't returned and we couldn't find out what was happening. The journalists in London were calling me to say that the meeting had ended and the HFEA had reached a decision. They were about to announce it at the press conference. My father rang the HFEA on my behalf. At this point I was too distracted to be capable of holding a coherent conversation. The HFEA's press secretary confirmed what the journalists were telling me, but said that they couldn't tell me what the decision was.

My father went ballistic. 'What do you mean, you're about to tell the whole world, but you can't tell my daughter first?'

They said they would speak to my solicitors, but they couldn't communicate directly with me.

It was 5 p.m. We made another call to my solicitors. 'Has Richard returned yet?'

'No.'

'It's Diane Blood. Is there anyone there who can help me?' I explained the situation.

'I'm sorry, everyone has left for the evening,' the receptionist apologised.

A few more irate phone calls to the HFEA later, we managed to

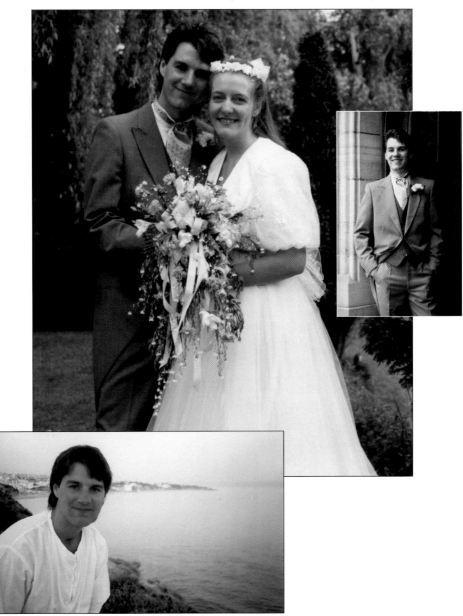

TOP: Me and Stephen on our wedding day, 11 May 1991.
(Photograph by Michael Penty)

TOP INSET: Stephen on our wedding day, 11 May 1991.
(Photograph by Michael Penty)

ABOVE: Stephen on our honeymoon in Albufeira, Portugal, May 1991.

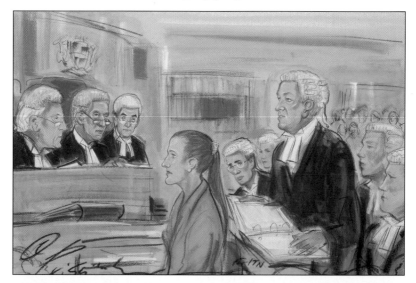

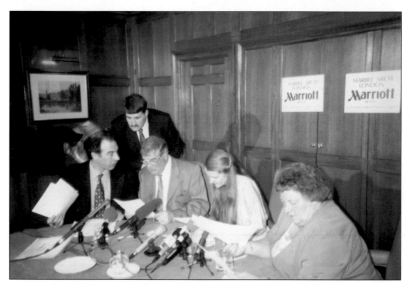

TOP: Court of Appeal, 13–15 January 1997.
From left to right: Lord Justice Waite, Lord Woolf M.R., Lord Justice Henry,
me, David Pannick QC and Dinah Rose (barristers for the HFEA), Lord
Lester of Herne Hill QC, Michael Fordham and Peter Duffy (my barristers)
(by Priscilla Coleman for Independent Television News)

ABOVE: The moment the fax that finally permitted export of Stephen's sperm
was received from the HFEA. This was taken while we were reading it, before
we realised that it gave me what I'd been asking for, on 27 February 1997.
From left to right: Richard Stein, Paul Plant, my father, me and my mother.

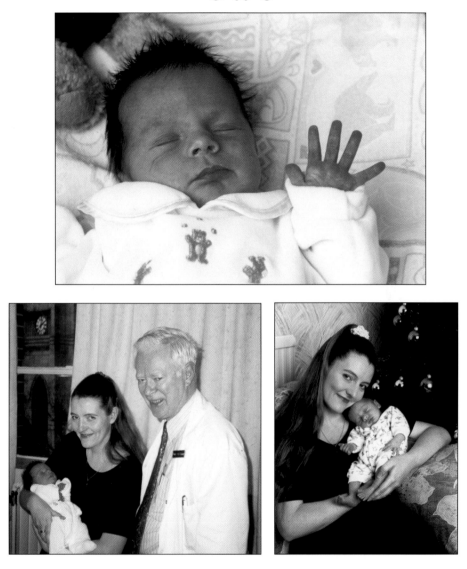

TOP: Liam, 24 December 1998. (Photograph by Andy Gallacher)

ABOVE LEFT: Liam and me with Professor Ian Cooke at the
Jessop Hospital for Women, 24 December 1998.

ABOVE RIGHT: Me and Liam, Christmas 1998.
(Photograph by Andy Gallacher)

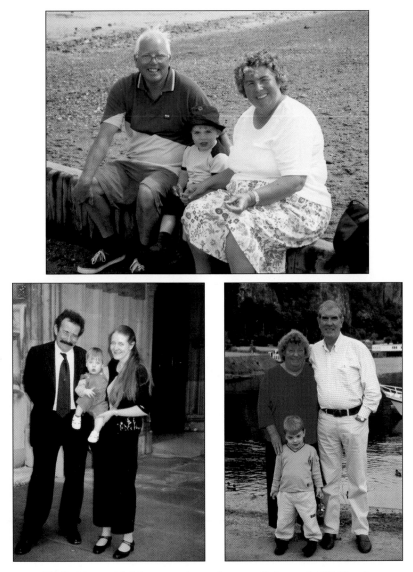

TOP: Liam with his paternal grandparents Brian and Gill Blood, Skegness, summer 2001.

ABOVE LEFT: Me and Liam with Professor Lord Winston outside the House of Lords, autumn 1999.

ABOVE RIGHT: Liam with his maternal grandparents Michael and Sheila McMahon, Belgium, October 2001.

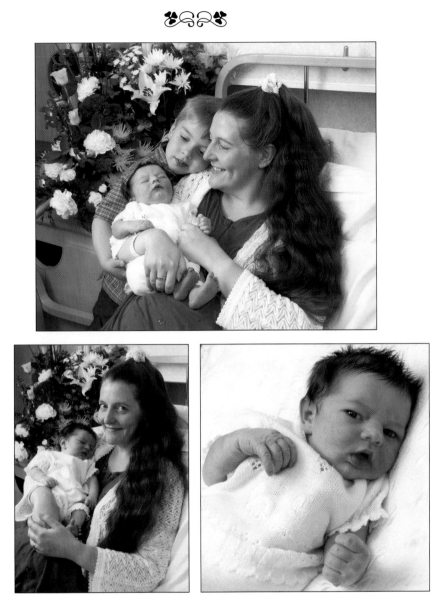

TOP: Liam, Joel and me, 18 July 2002.
(Photograph by Andy Gallacher)

ABOVE LEFT: Joel and me, 18 July 2002.
(Photograph by Andy Gallacher)

ABOVE RIGHT: Joel, 18 July 2002.
(Photograph by Andy Gallacher)

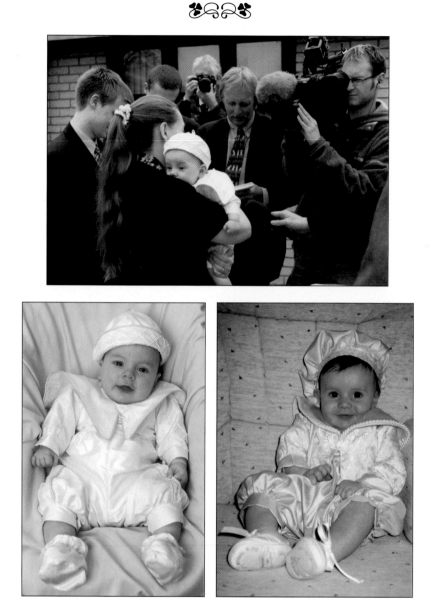

TOP: Liam's Baptism Day, 2 May 1999.

ABOVE LEFT: Liam on his Baptism Day, 2 May 1999.

ABOVE RIGHT: Joel on his Baptism Day, 27 October 2002.

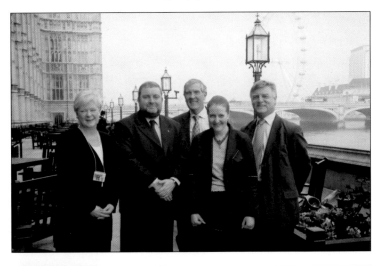

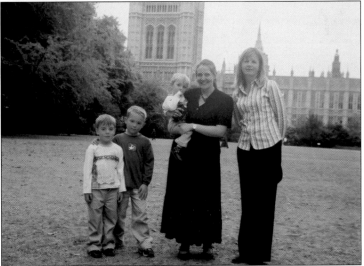

TOP: On the balcony at the House of Commons at the second reading
of Stephen McCabe's Human Fertilisation and Embryology
(Deceased Fathers) Bill, 28 March 2003. *From left to right*:
Sue Hayes (researcher for Stephen McCabe MP), Tony Clarke MP,
my father, me and Stephen McCabe MP.

ABOVE: Outside Westminster after the Human Fertilisation and Embryology
(Deceased Fathers) Bill finally completed its passage through Parliament,
18 September 2003. *From left to right*: Liam, Jonathan Tarbuck
(our co-litigant in our birth certificate court case), Joel,
me and Joanne Tarbuck (Jonathan's mother).

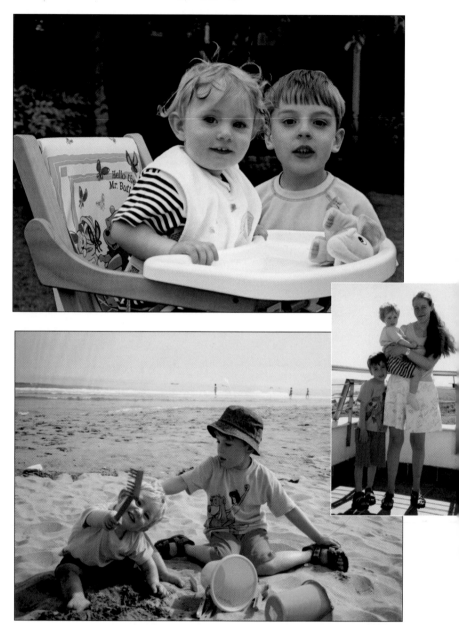

TOP: Liam and Joel at home in the garden, spring 2003.

ABOVE: Isla Canela in Spain: Liam and Joel on the beach in summer 2003 and (*inset*) the most recent photo of our family together at Easter 2004.

get an assurance that I would be informed, via my solicitors, before the announcement was made to the press. We explained that my solicitor's office had closed for the evening, but the HFEA said they still could not tell me direct. We offered my solicitor's home phone number, but the press had already given it to them. There was total confusion. By now the media in London were all seated at the conference waiting to hear the decision, and everyone was getting very frustrated. They all assumed that I must know, so they kept ringing me. We had to employ the ITN reporters who were with me to call and verify that I didn't.

Finally, my mother, who by this point was in tears, managed to get through to my dad. ITN had just broadcast that a decision was to be announced any minute and that it was expected to go in my favour. As ITN's inside information about the day's events had so far proved to be correct, she took this as extremely good news. Her tears were ones of joy.

The whole thing was getting ridiculous. My dad explained to the ITN reporters that, in view of the situation, he would have to take me up to their house so my family could be together. The cameras had already been set up in the office, but they could see my family's obvious distress and offered no protest. They said they would put the cameras away and follow us up in the van. They agreed to wait outside on my parents' drive.

My change of location was quickly relayed to the pack in London and to the numerous other reporters who, by now, were on their way up the M1 so they could be with me to record my reaction. The phones stopped ringing at work and started at my parents' house. The throng in London were still sitting with the HFEA waiting for the conference to begin. They were becoming increasingly agitated by the delay, but fortunately their anger was not channelled towards me. They knew that I was even more eager to know the result than they were. We had three phones ringing simultaneously: two mobiles and a landline. We were trying to juggle them and answer them all at once, hoping beyond hope that soon one of them would be my solicitor calling to say he was home.

Alas, the long-awaited call did not arrive, but eventually I received a new message via the media. 'Your solicitor is home and the HFEA have told him the result.'

The person on the other end of the line couldn't understand why I didn't know.

'Please will you tell everyone to stop ringing me. He won't be able to get through. The lines are constantly engaged.'

The message went back, but was ignored. No journalist could afford to let someone else know before they did and so the frustration continued. Another ring, another phone call answered. Another journalist. Another reporter. Until eventually . . .

'Diane. It's Richard.' My dad held out the phone and I took the call.

Richard's words were simply, 'I'm sorry.'

He offered no further explanation and I asked for none as I broke down into tears and handed the phone back to my dad.

My parents looked slightly bewildered. 'Diane, what's wrong?' They, as I, had expected the news to go for me and they could hardly make out my words as I collapsed down the wall, wailing, 'No, it's no.'

My dad spoke to Richard in the hope of getting further explanation. 'What were their reasons?'

Apparently, they hadn't been prepared to disclose them to him, saying that they would be given out at the press conference and then issued to ourselves in writing the following day.

Richard had pointed out that this was not acceptable and that they must tell us first. No reasons were forthcoming, but it seemed that events were to sort themselves out. Having already kept the press waiting for several hours, the HFEA had been forced to call off their press conference only moments before my solicitor had finally got through to me, so they wouldn't be telling anyone that evening after all.

The phones were still ringing, but we stopped answering them. The press recognised the difference and knew we knew. ITN knocked at the door. We kept the curtains closed and we tried to ignore them. I needed the racket to shut up. I was already being deafened by the piercing inner scream exploding in my head.

My dad went to the door and explained, 'She knows. It's not good. She needs some space. Please give us that before we talk to you.'

'Of course.'

They went back to the van.

Suddenly, I remembered. 'Gill, Stephen's mum. I haven't told her.'

I got on the phone straight away, but it was too late. The reporters who'd been camped outside her door had relayed the bad news.

The phones were still ringing. There was no escape and no time to grieve.

'Diane, you've got to talk to the press. You can cry later. Right now, you've got to go out there and fight.'

I knew my dad was right.

'OK, OK. Try and organise a conference for me, but the BBC are en route and still need time to get here.'

'How about eight o'clock?'

'All right. Go for eight.'

Within seconds, my dad was on the phone trying to organise the loan of the function room at The Innings; the landlady was happy to be of assistance. The word was passed around and the reporters removed themselves from the drive and went up to the pub to wait for me.

Eight o'clock had seemed to give me reasonable breathing space when we'd fixed the time, but in actual fact I had no time to prepare. My parents were on constant phone-answering duty. Some reporters were pleading for more time to get to Worksop. Others wanted to confirm the details of where to go.

If it hadn't been tragic, it would have been comical. Earlier that evening, they'd all been sitting in London waiting for the HFEA's conference to begin. It had eventually been called off and now they were all speeding north, trying to make it in time for mine. Same news, just a change of presenter and venue, and the minor issue of a few hundred miles in between.

We eventually escaped the house about half past eight, assured by the constant mobile-phone progress reports that most people would be there by the time we arrived. I still hadn't thought about what to say. To be honest, I was in a bit of a daze. It didn't seem real. More like watching a movie in which I could see myself act, yet I knew I wasn't present.

The pub car park was packed with satellite dishes and photographers. A runner from the BBC urged me to hurry upstairs to the function room. 'The news is at nine. We're on air in a few moments. We'll have to put you out virtually live. Do you think you can manage it?'

Manage it? It was all I could do to remember to breathe and just live through the next second, without caring about the practicalities of their programme editing.

'Yes, I'll be fine.'

My parents steered me through the pub doors. The wall of cameras and photographers rushed backwards in front of me. I'd grown used to them shouting directions, *Diane, this way . . . Look down the lens . . . Over here . . . Lift your head up.*

This time was different. No one said a word. Even the locals at the bar curtailed all conversation as I walked in through the door. Instead, they burst into applause. I could have cried. I was so grateful. When my husband first died, everyone always seemed to say the wrong thing. There are times when words are totally inadequate, but these strangers still let me know they supported me in the only way they could in those few seconds, as my parents, myself and the media entourage brushed past them and headed upstairs to the function room.

I actually smiled as I walked into the room. I was determined not to show how much they were getting me down. With the appeal in sight and preparation underway, there was no question of giving up, so I was quite surprised when journalists started to question whether I would, or even should, continue with the legal action. I was absolutely gutted by the day's events, but it had no bearing on the legal arguments we had prepared. I had been judged by the prosecution with no representative for the defence. A decision in my favour would have come as a huge relief and would have been very welcome, but it was not a substitute for a two-sided hearing in front of impartial judges. I reminded the reporters that this was merely an aside to the main action that had been declared and brought into the limelight by the HFEA. It was not another court case.

Instead, it now appeared to have been a cruel and pointless exercise. It had undermined my appeal for public donations and it had knocked my morale for six. I believed that its purpose had been to wear me down and, to an extent, it had succeeded. The pain it inflicted was almost unbearable. I felt as though I was dying by inches and I accused the HFEA of 'mental torture'. It was and still is the most graphic description I can think of for the anguish I was forced to bear.

I didn't sleep that night, but still the hours passed too quickly. There is something strangely calming about lying alone in a silent, darkened room. I didn't want the morning to come. Periodically, I found myself sobbing, but mostly I just lay staring into the emptiness. I really thought that I might be able to feel my husband's presence. I felt sure that his spirit would not leave me to cope with this alone, but I felt nothing. No magic strength. No Godly comfort. Just the workings of my own mind, churning things over and slowly sending the whole world sour.

If only I could stop my brain, I might be able to rest, but there was obviously going to be no respite. As I clearly couldn't forget about my troubles, I made a conscious decision to focus on my next plan of action. I think it must be something that was instilled in me at school. I really believed that, at the end of the day, it was all down to how much effort you put in. Work hard enough, and you can do the impossible. Fail, and you have only yourself to blame. I still had another chance. Next time, I'd just have to do better.

Thinking of the positive steps I might be able to take did help. At least it reminded me that the HFEA were not in control. In the cold light of day, I am not sure we can control our own destiny either, but it was a myth that helped me survive the night.

The following morning began with several radio interviews. The first was for Radio 4's *Today* programme. They had three guests: myself, Lord Winston and Dr Stuart Horner, the author of the BMA letter. After the interview, Lord Winston held on the phone line for a very quick word in private. 'You're doing OK. You're saying the right things. Just keep expressing your sadness and keep going.'

The encouragement was welcome. I wanted to talk for longer, but he had another appointment and had to hang up.

A few seconds later, I understood the rush to get off the phone. We were also all on the next programme together. And the one after that. Stuart Horner really upset me. Not because of his opinion but because he was so badly informed. His letter had claimed that, in the view of the BMA Medical Ethics Committee, 'whether the consent is in writing or given orally is irrelevant. The essential issue is the quality of that consent'. Previously, the BMA's spokesperson, Dr Stella Lowry, had issued a statement in which the BMA accepted that 'she has effectively got the consent of her husband'. But Stuart Horner continued, 'From the information which has been portrayed in the media, there is no evidence that Mr Blood had clearly thought through the issue and the full implications of a child being created after his death. Rather, it appears that he made a passing comment whose validity is difficult to evaluate in retrospect.' How could he say there was 'no evidence' when he hadn't even asked to see it? Before the first court case, I'd already been condemned by one organisation who didn't know the evidence and now this man was speaking on behalf of another group who hadn't examined the facts.

I complained about being given only a morning to reply to his letter. Stuart Horner pointed out, in his defence, that he had only been given something like a day to write it himself. This was interesting, partly because it was hardly enough time to seek the views of other members, but most importantly because the evidence later supplied to court claimed that his letter was unsolicited. When this transpired, I busied myself obtaining transcripts of the day's interviews to prove my point, but my solicitors wouldn't let me submit them as evidence. In the great scheme of things, they didn't think it was so important. I, on the other hand, felt most indignant about the whole episode.

When it appeared that Stuart Horner was losing the media battle on the specific nature of my late husband's oral consent for want of examining the actual facts, he switched to commenting that my case could have serious ramifications for consent regarding organ donation. He claimed that it could lead to a situation where a wife or husband would be able to donate their spouse's organs without their consent. This argument did, and still does, mystify me totally. On someone's death, it *is* the next of kin who is approached for permission to remove organs. This happens irrespective of the deceased's own opinion on the subject, although I'm sure most relatives would want to honour their loved one's wishes, where they were known. I tried pointing this out and asking interviewers for clarification of his point, as I was obviously missing something. Eventually I discovered that he meant that a spouse might ask for organs to be removed whilst the patient was still alive. I was taken aback by the stupidity of the idea. Why would any relative or doctor want to be doing that? Whatever happened to common sense?

There was more, but after just three short radio interviews I was exhausted and I'd had enough. I also had a couple of prearranged appointments for the day. The first was with Professor Cooke at the Jessop Hospital for Women. He'd arranged for me to begin seeing a specialist fertility counsellor at the hospital. The second was with a friend for lunch in Sheffield. I cancelled lunch and asked my dad to take me over to the Jessop. The mobiles kept on ringing whilst we were en route. We told everyone I was out of touch until lunchtime, which the journalists found very frustrating.

The switchboard had also been busy at the Jessop Hospital. As they were still holding the sperm, reporters were also seeking interviews with hospital representatives. I left my father with the mobiles and disappeared into the temporary sanctuary of the hospital. I was relieved to be sitting behind closed doors and to have a bit of respite from the commotion outside. I was unavailable. The Jessop Hospital was unavailable. The media never guessed where I was.

An hour or so later, with my sanity somewhat restored, I left feeling ready to face more interviews. Whilst I had been otherwise engaged, my dad had arranged that I'd do a couple of TV slots for the lunchtime news. They'd arranged to film me in Sheffield because that happened to be where I was at the time. We had to rush to make the deadline. We shot up to BBC Radio Sheffield, where they also have some TV studio facilities, and then straight down with the film crew to the Botanical Gardens, a public park, for a more aesthetically pleasing setting.

It seemed the news was gaining momentum, with more and more people being recruited to offer their opinion. Joe Ashton, my MP, had decided to join in, calling for the HFEA members to be sacked. One or two doctors also complained that, as members of the BMA, their views were not reflected by Dr Stuart Horner. Others decided to point out how ill I was looking, again offering up the idea that it might be best if I surrendered and gave up the fight. I'd had no sleep for two days and, due to lack of time and interest, no food either. It was hardly surprising that I didn't look my best, but, as a woman, I have to say I found it rather inconsiderate to be dragged onto TV and then told how dreadful I looked. I still cared – very slightly.

I did non-stop interviews for the rest of the day. In the afternoon, I called my second press conference in 24 hours at The Innings to try to abate some of the interest from the day before. I had thought it would only be a very short conference, just to answer a few outstanding questions, but, in the middle of it, my solicitor called on the mobile to say he'd just been faxed the HFEA's reasons for refusing to allow export. The reporters hung on while my dad went home to fetch the fax and they gave me the time and privacy for a quick mobile phone call to my solicitor, so that we could discuss their implications.

There were four points detailed in their document:

> 1. Parliament has enacted a careful code allowing for posthumous use of sperm only if specific requirements are met. In particular, there is a clear requirement for the written and effective consent of a man, after he has had the opportunity to receive counselling and after he has had a proper opportunity to consider the implications of a posthumous birth. These important requirements were not satisfied in this case.
>
> 2. The Authority does not think that it would be right to allow Mrs Blood to export the sperm to avoid the specific requirements which prevent her from using the sperm in this country. The Authority noted that Mrs Blood has no prior connection with any country to which she wishes to export the sperm.
>
> 3. In the context of the use of genetic material the Authority considers that any consent should be given in clear and formal terms by the person himself or herself and that the Authority is reluctant to seek to identify a person's wishes from the evidence of another person.
>
> 4. The Authority also bore in mind that Mr Blood had not given any consideration, let alone consent, to the export of his sperm to another country.

It was nothing we hadn't heard before in one form or another. The legal team were pleased. They thought it strengthened our case that the HFEA couldn't come up with anything else.

I was pleased that, at that moment, at least the waiting TV and press presence gave me some way of answering back, 'But they haven't commented on the evidence. The question they had to ask was *whether to permit export in the absence of written consent and the formalities required by domestic law?* So how can it be a sensible answer to not allow export simply because I don't have those things which were the very reason for the question in the first place. They'd used a lot of words, but essentially all they'd done was repeat the question and refuse to look beyond it.

The journalists who were present appeared to think the reasons were as daft as I did.

I seemed to be gaining sympathy. By around 5 p.m., Stuart Horner had changed his tune. In the last interview we both did, he told the reporter that all he had heard all day was that they hadn't looked at the evidence. He offered no criticism of my situation, but instead merely said, 'so send us the evidence'.

I would gladly have done so, had the damage not already been done.

My final interview of the day was to be with *Calendar* news in Leeds. Again my dad came with me, but they sent a taxi to fetch us. I did a couple of radio interviews from the mobile phone on the way, which was interesting because the car was noisy and the driver kept turning the radio on. The interviewers wanted us to stop, but we couldn't because we didn't have time. I could hardly hear and, with all the racket going off in the background, I must have sounded pretty dreadful. Still, at least no one can say you look bad on the radio.

I didn't make it for that last appointment, or rather I did, but I was a fraction too late. We hit heavy traffic and the programme was on air before we arrived. We phoned in with details of our progress and someone met us at the door. We ran hell for leather along the corridors up to the studio. I shed my coat and bag along the way, calling to my dad, who was trailing behind, to pick them up. We made it into the studio just in time for the closing minutes of the programme. It was too late to squeeze in an interview, so they apologised to their audience that I hadn't made it and, after a quick aside confirming that I'd pre-record something for Monday's programme, promised that they would be speaking to me after the weekend.

We then caught our breath and recorded the piece for Monday's news. I was relieved the day's work was over.

CHAPTER 13

The House of Lords debates our predicament

Things were looking up. The evidence for the appeal was coming along nicely. We'd employed another barrister, Peter Duffy, to work solely on the European Community law angle of the case, and with the reasons for refusing export now in writing and submitted in evidence by the HFEA, we were confident that no court would view them as reasonable justification. The constant angst that I had lived with ever since the case began almost started to subside, even though I knew I was still a long way from success.

Lord Winston called to cheer me further. He'd been trying to get a Bill through the House of Lords to change the law, supported by Baroness Warnock. They had a date for the second reading at the beginning of December. He invited me and my family down for the debate.

In the meantime, *Heart of the Matter* (with the film made by the former HFEA member Robert Snowdon) was due to be recorded the next week and broadcast before the Lords debate. We needed bad publicity right now like we needed a hole in the head and I was still terrified by the programme. Lord Winston and Baroness Warnock had apparently agreed to go on and speak for my side, whilst, in addition to Robert Snowdon, the editor of a medical ethics magazine and a Christian author were appearing for the opposition. I still didn't think they should be talking about me 'behind my back' and, with the HFEA decision cruelly going against me, I decided I couldn't afford to pussyfoot around any longer. As I couldn't prevent it from being broadcast altogether, I called and volunteered to record a short interview with Joan Bakewell, the presenter, to be inserted into the middle of the programme, and then agreed to appear in the latter half of the debate.

This format was accepted and we recorded the programme the following week. My dad drove me down south to arrive at the studio in plenty of time. The programme participants gathered together in one room. I was delighted to meet Baroness Warnock for the first time. I also tried to make polite conversation with some of those who were appearing against me, but it was a total charade which quickly degenerated into an argument on the topic we were supposed to be saving for the programme. The atmosphere was venomous.

Joan Bakewell came in to discover us in the middle of a heated exchange on the topic of the first Gulf War. Before going to Iraq, many soldiers deposited sperm for use by their wives in case they didn't return. This was allegedly encouraged by the army, not only because of the possibility of death but also because the men might fear castration if they were caught by the enemy. With the benefit of hindsight and knowledge of the subsequent birth-defect problems in veterans' children, to my mind, it might just have been a good idea anyway, but I don't suppose that one figured in anyone's imagination at the time.

Grateful to be given a reason to escape, I followed Joan down into the studio to record my interview. She checked a few details with me, asked me to keep it simple and not resort to legal-speak and then off we went. I thought I made a reasonable job of answering her questions and was pleased I'd managed to get out most of what I'd wanted to say. I included my views on marriage and that I considered us 'of one flesh'. The only point I hadn't managed to convey was that I could have used the sperm of an anonymous donor, even one who was dead, and yet not that of my own husband. I made a mental note to find some way of getting this into the debate later.

Next, it was everyone else's turn in the studio. My dad and I watched on a TV monitor whilst Robert Snowdon's film was played and everyone watched it for the first time. The participants were then led onto the set one at a time. My opposition went on armed with a whole bunch of legal papers, which they plonked on the table in front of them.

Joan Bakewell interceded, 'First of all, let me say that I am concerned about all these papers.'

Not half as concerned as I was. She was only halfway through the sentence when I flew into the studio and onto the set, determined to make sure they stopped filming. A huge row ensued between myself, Robert Snowdon and the man from the medical ethics magazine. One of the items they had brought was the HFEA's Code of Practice, which they wished to demonstrate clearly states that a man's sperm cannot be used without his consent following his death.

This, to me, showed the complete and dangerous lack of understanding about what my legal case was actually about. I didn't dispute how clearly this new Code of Practice made the point, but it was published in December 1995, eight months after my husband had died. Presumably the reason for its inclusion was precisely because of my situation. The previous Code had included no such reference and that was the whole reason for the judicial review. We had applied within three months of the new Code being issued to make a move to strike the new point on account of what we alleged to be its illegality. I tried to explain, but everyone was too busy shouting to listen. I argued that I hadn't come here to face another court case, and if they were going to quote ill-researched facts from legal documents, I was going. I wasn't alone in my threat to take my bat and ball and disappear off home. My verbal assailants also got up and began to leave the studio.

Joan Bakewell looked on the scene with the quiet calm of one who has some experience of caring for unruly children. 'When you've all finished, I believe this is my programme and I should know the type of things we do and don't include. Legal papers aren't among them. Now, shall we get rid of them and start again?'

The papers went, we all stayed and the rest of the programme passed without incident. In fact, in the end, I was rather glad I'd participated, as I thought it came out quite well and hoped it might help with support for Lord Winston's Bill.

The opinion polls were still tipped 90 per cent in my favour by the time we went to the House of Lords on 5 December. In fact, if anything, the treatment I'd received following the HFEA's decision against me had strengthened public support for my cause. I'd received huge amounts of sympathetic mail, a *Calendar* news telephone poll had drawn their highest ever number of respondents, 24,000, and I'd had one particularly generous anonymous offer of financial help. That took a pretty big weight off my mind.

Three of us travelled down to London on the train: my dad, Gill (my late husband's mother) and myself. Again, there was huge media interest and we had to weave our way through the cameras to gain entrance to Westminster.

The debate was markedly different to the one we had attended in the House of Commons. Some spoke for me, some against, and some made their point quite eloquently without making it totally clear which side they were on. Altogether, it seemed a much more sensible and dignified affair than the Commons.

I was touched when Lord Winston said my affidavit, laying out the facts of my situation for the court, had moved him to tears because he believed 'that a fundamental injustice was being done'. This, he told the House, was despite the fact that at the time he had never met me, it was two o'clock in the morning and he was not already in an emotional state as he was 'quite tired' and 'about to go to bed'.

Baroness Warnock, in particular, made an extremely well-reasoned speech, clarifying many of the points which had been misrepresented in the past. It was particularly interesting that she pointed out that she herself had been born after her father's death, so she was hardly likely to believe that posthumous children suffered psychological problems as a result.

As usual, factual inaccuracies made me want to scream out the truth, even though some of them were of little relevance. Lord Ashbourne claimed that I was 'tragically widowed at 30'. I wasn't. I was 28. Hansard will stand long after I am dead and gone, and these people were casually rewriting my life history. What was more upsetting were mistakes that also referred to my husband. He was no longer here to correct the record. Lord Kilbracken said, 'We know the couple had been married, happily we believe, for a considerable period – seven or eight years – and yet no children resulted.' He questioned therefore why we hoped artificial methods might be effective where 'normal intercourse and/or assisted intercourse' had failed. I wanted to scream out that we'd only been married for three and a half years when we'd started trying for a baby and there was nothing wrong with our fertility. It was just that we'd only had a month or so of attempting to conceive a child before Steph had died.

One or two times I looked across at Gill to see tears in her eyes. 'They're talking about my son,' she explained, as though she had to.

'I know,' I volunteered. I tried to look on the positive side. 'He wanted his name to go down in history, but I bet he never thought he'd end up in Hansard.'

We both exhaled breath and gave a half-nervous smile. I was glad Gill had been spared the ordeal of sitting through the House of Commons debate. If this one upset her, I don't think she'd have survived the former.

I think I was having to become partially immune to it all. There was just one point which grated on my soul. It was the strong opposition offered up by the Bishop of Oxford. He commented that, 'A great many young men die every year and leave a great number of grieving wives, girlfriends and parents. It would be entirely understandable if a high percentage of them wanted to carry something of the person they loved into the future in the form of a child.' He totally misunderstood my reasons for wanting Steph's child.

This misunderstanding was then amplified by a statement made by Lord Habgood. Lord Habgood pointed out that legally 'death dissolves a marriage', and he worried about 'the pressures to deny death or to circumvent it'. At the end of his speech, he returned to the point, 'Doctors can do wonderful things in preserving the living. But I hope that we shall not let them persuade us into still further attempts to preserve the potency of the dead. I am one of those who believes that death is not the end. Because I believe that, I believe that we must let the dead go in order to find them again. That is why my Christian conviction works in this instance against the attractions of immediate compassion.'

It is very difficult to explain, but these comments ate away at the foundations of my faith in the established Church. I am a Christian, too, and yet the implication was that I couldn't be because he assumed I saw things differently. I, too, believed my husband had found eternal life in heaven. My desire to have

Steph's children predated and had nothing to do with his death. I wasn't trying to bring him back. I wanted our child, a unique God-given creation. At that point, it seemed as though I didn't have a lot left. Through it all, I'd just about managed to cling onto my faith. Now, I felt like I'd just been excommunicated.

Thankfully, when the debate was over and we were on our way out of the door, another bishop came to my spiritual rescue. He explained that, although there had been three bishops present at the debate, only one was allowed to speak. The other two had been surprised at the stance taken and wanted to offer their support. 'We don't all think like that, you know. Some of us think that love continues beyond the grave.'

I was grateful to know that I didn't stand alone and against the whole Christian population. It had hit a very disturbing and dangerous nerve. One week, as I left church, a woman from our congregation had handed me a prayer card entitled, 'An old woman's prayer'. I read it. It was about departed loved ones and having the grace not to complain. But I wasn't an old woman. I'd temporarily considered having a slanging match with her in the church doorway, but a voice told me to forgive her, as she didn't understand, so I simply handed back the card without saying a word and gave her a hug for trying to help. Personally, I thought that only God could pull me through this unscathed and I had no doubts that what I was doing was right and according to His will. I had even taken comfort from the many Christians who had written to me pointing out various passages in the Bible.

'Take a look at this chapter or that verse,' they told me. 'It's God's special word for you.'

Luke 18, the Parable of the Persistent Widow, also held special significance in my heart. After the HFEA's decision to refuse export, many had said it was time to end the fight. One woman had written into a newspaper saying she was sick of hearing about it. That particularly hurt. If she was sick of it, imagine how I felt. Of course, I consulted God for His opinion. The following Sunday, I was flicking through the Bible at church. It fell open on the page containing this specific chapter. Apart from being particularly apt in its subject matter, it tells of how God answers the prayers of those who keep asking. In the case of this parable, the judge grants justice to the persistent widow because he fears she will eventually wear him out by repeatedly asking. I don't think God could have made Himself much plainer if He'd appeared before me in person. I just didn't feel equipped to take on the Church as well as everyone else.

The Lords debate had ended with a vote over whether the Bill should be allowed to proceed to the Committee stage. The motion was carried and there was a promise by the Parliamentary Under-Secretary of State for the Department of Health, Baroness Cumberlege, to hold a review into the present law on consent. Sheila McLean, a professor from Glasgow University, was named to write the report. It appeared to be a similar tactic to that employed at the end of the Commons debate.

Here, look, the Government's going to do something. Now be satisfied, shut up and stop pursuing the Bill through Parliament.

In fact, this was more or less the summary offered by Baroness Cumberlege after the debate. Lord Winston introduced us. She was very pleasant and said she hoped I was happy with the Government's response. Even though she acknowledged that it would probably come too late for me, she said that it might help others. She also expressed her wishes that Lord Winston would now feel able to drop his Bill.

He paused slightly, as though considering it and then continued, 'Do you know, I don't think I will.'

I smiled. Of course I wasn't satisfied with what the Government had offered. I wanted something done about my problem – now – not some lame promise to look into it at some unspecified time in the future.

Lord Lester joined us. He had been in the Lords for the debate, but he hadn't spoken, due to his role as my QC. He was also invited to have dinner with Lord Winston's party. Everyone milled around in the lobby for a while, passing various opinions on how things had gone and on what to say to the awaiting press.

As we were actually having dinner within the building, there was no reason to go outside, but we decided to appease the mob by nipping outdoors and speaking to them briefly before returning to enjoy the rest of the evening. I thought it a bit unfair to leave them hanging around all night, wondering if I was ever going home. The reporters wanted to know what I thought of Baroness Cumberlege's promise of a review. Suddenly, everyone seemed to expect me to be an expert in parliamentary procedures, when really the reporters would have had far more idea than I. I thought it might be a lot more useful if they told me what they thought, but they wouldn't be drawn on the subject. I said my piece about pinning all my hopes on the Court of Appeal and everyone was happy.

With the debate and the media out of the way, I could now relax. Lord Winston's wife and son had also joined us. It was an extremely pleasant evening. Not everyone gets to dine in the House of Lords and I felt very privileged.

I was still being inundated with requests to appear on other programmes. For the most part, I'd declined, but then one came up which was too good to miss. I was asked to do a short interview on *Breakfast with Frost*. Being a political news programme, it would be watched by the target audience I most wanted to reach.

My dad again drew the short straw to drive me down to the BBC's London studios. We were thinking of going that night and staying over in a hotel. The programme was being recorded live the following morning and I had to be there very early. Before we made our arrangements, we still had to wait for them to call me back and confirm who would be appearing to present the case against me.

As the day wore on, it became apparent that they had a problem. They'd been through everyone they could think of and all had refused.

'No one wants to argue against you any more,' the programme researchers told me.

After everything I'd been through, particularly with *Heart of the Matter*, it was like being told that I'd won the media war. Did this mean that when I next refused to do a programme, I would no longer have to worry about them making it anyway but from the opposing perspective? I was pleased, but at the same time a little disappointed, as it meant they couldn't really have me on the programme. They wouldn't put out a one-sided argument.

Late that night, they called me back. Sir David Frost would still really like me to appear on the programme and there was one way of putting over an apparently unbiased message. The interviewer could play devil's advocate, putting over questions from the opposition's point of view. He hadn't really wanted to do this, but they suggested that, as I knew the opposing argument as well as my own, I might like to be professional enough to write my own questions for him to put to me. They would obviously be checked for suitability, but it was rather a novel situation. Now I got to be my own prosecution and defence, just as the HFEA had been in the meeting on export. The difference was I had only two to three minutes of air time in which to do it and I still had an independent jury. It's a shame that *Breakfast with Frost* didn't have the power to alter my future in the same way as the HFEA's meeting.

By this time, it was too late to leave that night, so we had to get up and leave at some unearthly hour of the morning. It was still dark when we arrived, although the deafening alarm that was clattering through the studios at the time was enough to waken anyone.

'What on earth is that?' I asked.

They explained that it was the Royal Death alarm. No one had died. It was just a practice. They told me that when the alarm went off (which at the time everyone presumed would be for the Queen Mother's death), they had to immediately abandon the normal schedule and switch to sombre music. It never occurred to anyone that next time it sounded for real it would actually be for Diana, Princess of Wales. I even heard later from an Australian film crew that their station had picked up the drill I had heard and mistakenly announced the Queen Mother's death. It just goes to show how dangerous it is to jump to conclusions before knowing the facts.

I was shown to a dressing-room where I could get changed, write my questions and consider the answers. It was all quite leisurely, as we'd arrived in good time. As usual, there were a fair few politicians on the programme, and Esther Rantzen was also appearing. We met them in the Green Room, the backstage (or rather back-studio) waiting room, in between interviews. We had a better opportunity to talk when we all sat down to a cooked breakfast together after the programme had finished.

It was interesting meeting the politicians. I tried to pick their brains for any better solutions on how to go about changing the law or simply fixing my own problem. Esther Rantzen was also an extremely interesting and considerate woman. To be honest, I don't think anyone there that morning could understand what all the fuss was about. Esther Rantzen thought I should just get the SAS to go and 'nick the sperm' for me. She didn't see it as stealing, just reclaiming what was rightfully mine. Everyone agreed that I should just take the sperm out of Britain and go to 'some civilised country'. I got the impression that I would have no shortage of willing accomplices and plenty of people prepared to campaign on my behalf, so I wouldn't get prosecuted afterwards. It would certainly get the Government out of the jam with people calling to change a law that no one wanted to be discussed.

Of course, people had suggested before that I should steal the sperm. I'd even had a phone call out of the blue which had offered assistance from an expert in animal husbandry, who could store the sperm correctly should I manage to procure it. Plenty of others had called me with details of how to self-inseminate, but I might need IVF and I could just imagine what the Belgians would have thought if I'd suddenly turned up at their clinic without the proper documentation.

Oh, here's my husband's sperm. It's all a bit hush-hush, but will you still treat me even though I didn't obtain it legally?

I don't think it would have gone down well. Stealing it would also be easier said than done. Steph's sperm was stored under a codename to prevent easy identification. I have to admit I'm rather glad it was, as I was also worried that someone who opposed me might steal or destroy it themselves. Also, I had genuine reservations about being dishonest, as well as faith that justice would prevail. I had once jokingly asked my barrister, Michael Fordham, if he'd be able to save me from prosecution if I stole Steph's sperm. He laughed and jested about possibly getting off on the grounds of mental health, but commented that, if I broke the law myself, I could hardly ask the law to help me. I knew that and I believed in the Court of Appeal.

At the end of the meal, phone numbers were exchanged in case anyone could help me set up meetings with politicians I wanted to speak to. I never actually used any of them. I would have, if my back had been against the wall, but at this point I had every reason to trust that I was going to get there via the routes we already had in place.

CHAPTER 14

The Appeal

With my general feeling of optimism and the appeal scheduled to commence on 13 January, Christmas 1996 was almost bearable. It wasn't long to wait and the preparations were in hand and moving along as scheduled. My case was still being featured in the papers and I received good luck cards from members of the public, which I dotted in amongst the Christmas cards dangling from the units in my lounge. Of course, I still really missed Steph, but this year I certainly didn't feel alone.

In the run up to Christmas I went to take a seasonal wreath to Stephen's grave. It was bitter at the cemetery. It's an exposed spot and it always seems cold there, even in the middle of the summer. I wanted to enjoy the peace and tell Stephen not to worry, that we would win the court case and that I'd soon be able to try for his baby. I hope he got the message because I never actually had time for the words to form. People kept approaching me, offering their good wishes and support. They told me about their own loved ones whom they had come to visit. Some were recently bereaved; many were visiting husbands or wives who had died long, long ago. I wondered about all these souls in heaven and smiled as I thought perhaps they would offer comfort to Steph, as their relatives did to me. Eventually the crisp air prevented me from lingering beside the grave any longer. I found a convenient gap between the stream of well-wishers and left.

Christmas Day was split between my own parents (for lunch) and

Stephen's family (for tea). We also found time to listen to a radio broadcast, which was on just after lunchtime, about my case. I had done a short pre-recorded piece for it before the festivities started. I thought it rather a bizarre subject for Christmas Day, but then again I'm not in charge of scheduling. It was pretty much the usual stuff.

'Wouldn't it be better to give up?' they asked.

I knew that many members of the public and media, even those who supported my moral stance, believed I wouldn't win. I had to point out that they were not qualified to give a legal opinion.

Clare Dyer, the reporter from *The Guardian* who'd first interviewed me, was also on the programme. She decided to have a go at my appearance. She didn't like my long hair and generally didn't think I paid much attention to myself. Last time I'd seen her, she was jetting off for a shopping trip to New York to top up her wardrobe. On a restricted budget, I was really struggling for clothes. Before the first court case, I'd had to go out and buy three suits, as I didn't previously possess any. I'd worn one on each day and I'd subsequently worn them for TV appearances and the debates in the Houses of Commons and Lords. Not that many occasions really, but it appeared as though I'd worn them to death because they kept repeating the same old footage over and over on TV. With another three days of court and public scrutiny, I would have to buy some more. Why was I being judged on the way I looked? Clare Dyer may well have been right, but what relevance did it have? It was Christmas. I had to be careful with money. The experience I'd had to endure over the past year and eight months was enough to make anyone look dreadful. At that particular time, on that particular day, I did care, even though in my more rational moments I knew I shouldn't.

Money and stress were not the only barriers to conformity in my new world. It was a culture thing, too, and perhaps partly my personality. I liked long hair and have never really followed fashion. If I'd gone to New York, I wouldn't have known which shops to go in anyway. I'd progressed from dining out at the local pub, 'two meals for a fiver', to dining in the House of Lords. I didn't know how I should behave, but I was doing my best and being myself. Maybe that was my main problem, in the eyes of my critics. Then again, if they could mould me into the woman they'd rather I was, I wouldn't have been the kind of person to take issue with authority in the first place.

With Christmas over, the final preparations began for the court appearance. Our skeleton argument was written and had been submitted to the court and to the HFEA. It was pretty impressive and I knew we had a good case.

Basically, our three points of issue were the same as they had been at the first hearing.

In our document, we described them as follows:

> The Construction Issue – What is the meaning of the statutory exception regarding treatment for a couple 'together'?
>
> The Domestic Scrutiny Issue – Does the refusal to allow export of the sperm meet domestic standards of substantive review?
>
> The European Scrutiny Issue – Is that refusal consistent with EC Law?

The difference was that this time we had put a lot more work into the European side of the argument. Also, in case all else failed, we had a couple of new points on my best claim to ownership of the sperm. Since preparing our arguments for the first hearing, we discovered a judgement had recently been passed on a new relevant case. It was about a pickled brain, of all things. North Tyneside Health Authority had destroyed a pickled brain belonging to the Plaintiff's deceased relative. In that particular case, the health authority had won. The next of kin had no right to damages for the loss of the brain, but the judge made it clear in his *obiter dicta* (a spoken aside to a judgement which is not legally binding, but may nonetheless be taken into account) that the reason for this was because the brain was 'of no practical use'. It therefore followed that, as Stephen's sperm was of practical use whilst it was still frozen, I would have a right to ownership.

The other case was a 1993 Court of Appeal judgement from the USA. As such, it did not have a direct bearing on the English courts, but it could help to influence them. I couldn't remember my legal team mentioning it before, but maybe they had and just chose to give it more prominence for the Court of Appeal. The Appellant, Deborah Hecht, had won. In that case, the subject matter was frozen sperm, just the same as in mine. It was ruled that the sperm could constitute 'property' for the purposes of probate. What was even more noteworthy about this case, as far as we were concerned, was its conclusion regarding the absence of any public policy against posthumous insemination of a partner.

We thought we'd got everything ready and then immediately before the court case two more welcome articles were published. One was a letter by Sir Douglas Black, an eminent retired physician and former Government Chief Scientist and President of the BMA. On 9 January, he wrote in my support and accused the HFEA of 'corporate tyranny'. The other article, by Dr Kamal Ahuja, had been deliberately timed to be released just before my hearing. It concerned another woman who'd just been successfully impregnated with her husband's sperm, following treatment with ICSI (intracytoplasmic sperm injection, where a single sperm is injected into the egg) after his death. The treating clinic believed it to be the first case of posthumous insemination using this particular method of treatment. This woman had faced none of my legal problems because she had written consent, but it helped reiterate the real legal issue as being consent, not posthumous insemination per se.

Each of these events sent the media into a new frenzy and I had to work out how to answer the questions they posed. The latter article we decided to use in evidence. We obtained some copies of the *British Medical Journal*, where it had been published, to hand up to the judges. Now we really had to be ready.

For various reasons, from Stephen's family, only his mother Gill could attend the appeal hearing. She travelled down with us and we all stayed in a hotel. Stephen's former work colleagues who'd helped form the Stephen Blood Baby Appeal met up with us in London.

Mine was the first case to be heard after the Christmas break so, thankfully, as with my lower court hearing, I didn't have any worries about it not starting on schedule, but I was as nervous as anything. The night before it commenced, I didn't sleep a wink.

We ran the familiar gauntlet of the photographers at the front door and met up with everyone inside the Royal Courts of Justice, but before entering the Court of Appeal. Everyone seemed in a reasonably elevated mood, if a little tense. Michael Fordham, my barrister, revealed that he hadn't slept the previous night either. My QC couldn't understand our reports of insomnia. He was the one who had to do all the talking and, for my part, I didn't have to do a thing. Besides which, he always took sleeping tablets before a big case. He tried to persuade me to go and see a show that night, to take my mind off things. I wasn't convinced about the idea. I didn't think I'd be able to concentrate.

We watched as the files and papers were wheeled into the court on big barrows. There were tons of them. We joked that we knew that at least one of the judges had read most of the papers, as he'd called my solicitors that morning to report one of the pages missing from his bundle. The offending page was numbered a hundred and something. They were A4 pages. That means that just to get that far, without reading any asides, would mean having read approximately the same amount of information as that contained in this book this far. I hope that judges read faster than I do, otherwise they'd never get the job done. I felt rather sorry for them, with the amount of work it entailed, but, nonetheless, I would have felt cheated if they hadn't read all the files from cover to cover.

Ruth Deech, the chairwoman from the HFEA, arrived shortly before the court doors were opened, as did the HFEA's legal team. We soon filed into the room and took our places. It was a more modern courtroom than the one in which the first hearing had been held: much lighter, more airy and not so oppressive. The bench, reporters' gallery and any shelves in the room were made of light oak. One side of the room was decked with books. The other side, behind the area where the reporters sat, there were large windows. As at the first hearing, I sat right at the front, with my father and Richard Stein, my solicitor. Counsel for both sides were behind me. My mother sat with Gill further back in the court, where the seats were comfier and a bit less pew-like. The reporters were to my left, sitting at right angles to the rest of the court. Unlike the first hearing, they were not in my line of view when looking towards the judges, so it was easier to forget their presence. The all- important court clock was, however, positioned in clear view. It was fixed to the left-hand wall, just in front of the bench. Having learnt to fear the passage of time at the first hearing, the sight of it now filled me with the same kind of dread as the clock in a school exam.

The court rose for the entrance of the three judges: The Right Honourable The Lord Woolf, Master of the Rolls, Lord Justice

Henry and Lord Justice Waite. The court was in session, Lord Lester, my QC, rose to his feet and the clock began to tick.

There was less of a preamble to the case than there had been at the first hearing because, by now, everyone knew the basic facts. What we put forward were points of law: basically just going through our skeleton argument and expanding on it. Immediately the hearing seemed to be going better than the first one. The judges asked questions, so you knew they had understood what was put before them. Maybe it was just a difference of approach, but it felt much better.

First we went through the evidence to show that treating me with the sperm accorded with Stephen's wishes, even though, in court, none of this had ever been disputed by the HFEA. Then we moved on to why it could be classified as being in my husband's best interests. This 'best interest' test was important because, in common law, it is the measure which gives a doctor authority to act when the patient is unable or incapable of giving consent on their own behalf. For one part, this involved contrasting the opinions of the two expert witnesses, Professor Lord Winston on my behalf and Dr Shenfield (who, as I previously mentioned, was actually a paid member of the HFEA's staff) on their behalf. Dr Shenfield took a narrow interpretation of 'best interests', seeing it only as treatment which could be said to be a 'life-saving measure'. We demonstrated how courts in the past had taken a wider view. One of the cases we cited regarded the sterilisation of a mentally incapacitated adult woman, which was held to be in her 'best interests'. There were other cases too, say where a patient was alive but in a coma from which they would be extremely unlikely to ever regain consciousness. In that instance, it could be in their 'best interests' to turn off the life-support machine, even though this is obviously the opposite to a life-saving measure.

We also used the evidence of Stephen's conversation with me regarding posthumous insemination as justification for obtaining the sperm by reason of anticipatory consent. Even our wedding vows were quoted, and it was pointed out that it was unusual that we had deliberately chosen the somewhat archaic version that placed greater emphasis on procreation than the more modern text. Lord Lester, my QC, had said that he hoped I appreciated this, as, being a Jew, it was against his religion to mention Christ so many times. In fact, it was also blasphemous for many of the court.

Apparently, Lord Woolf MR was also Jewish, as too were my solicitor, Lord Winston, David Pannick QC and Dinah Rose (barristers for the HFEA), and Ruth Deech herself. Regardless of this, I don't suppose anyone's religious convictions stopped them from taking on board our point.

Next we moved on to the statute. We were making good time. It was going much better than the first hearing, but it was still emotionally wearing and I was relieved when we broke for lunch. We were quite cheerful, though, and after a short break, I felt reasonably well equipped to cope with round two of the day.

Our case for treatment in the UK relied on showing that Stephen and I were being 'treated together' (what we had termed the construction issue). The HFEA said that we could not be 'treated together' because, sadly, my husband was no longer here. Based on a normal understanding of English, this sounds pretty sensible at first glance, but we aimed to show that existing legal authority, as well as discussions contained in the White Paper (issued prior to the Act) and Hansard, indicated otherwise.

The only existing legal authority on the point of treatment 'together' was a case regarding disputed parentage. A man deposited sperm but then split with his wife before she was inseminated with the sperm. They were still regarded as falling within the treatment 'together' exception, so the man was deemed to be the father of the child. The court regarded the man's treatment as the removal of his sperm. It was immaterial that he was no longer present or even supportive by the time his sperm was used. 'Together' was not seen as an indication of physical proximity, but of the commencement of a joint enterprise. We argued that my husband and I had also commenced a joint enterprise to have a child. We were trying for a family naturally at the time of his death and we had also been 'together' as husband and wife at the time of the removal of his sperm, whilst he was still alive.

Naturally, the HFEA saw things differently. To them, treatment 'together' connoted the insemination of a woman with the sperm of a man (husband, partner or even just a known donor helping his female friend) who is alive at the time of insemination. This, basically, was the point we disputed in their new Code of Practice, issued in December 1995. It read as follows:

9.20 Insemination of a woman using her husband's or partner's sperm, while he is alive, is not regulated by the Human Fertilisation and Embryology Act 1990.

9.21 Insemination of a woman at a licensed centre using her late husband's or partner's sperm is regulated under the Act. For this to take place the man must have given consent to the posthumous use of his sperm to treat the woman. The law would regard this as treatment using the sperm of a donor . . .

One of our main points of contention with this was that, if correct, it made nonsense of one of the provisions set out in the 1990 Act. It was subsections 28(6) a&b which dealt specifically with paternity in cases of posthumous insemination. Parliament drew two distinct categories; in neither case would the deceased be regarded as father of the child. The first category was where the man had given consent. The second was where he had not. We therefore proposed that Parliament had expressly contemplated a second category of man whose sperm could be used after his death but who remained outside the written consent provisions. The only way this could possibly occur was if treatment 'together' could continue after the man's death.

In answer to this, the HFEA submitted an alternative. They proposed that the subsection may have been included to deal with the consequences of mistakes, where a child had already been created and someone had slipped through the net. This really hurt. Once again, I felt the twist of the knife protruding from my stomach. Why couldn't they have just let me slip through the net?

The trickiest area we had to overcome was the provisions laid down for storage within the Act. Storage required written consent in all cases. There were no exceptions for treatment 'together'. We had a number of different angles on this, but what was so uplifting about the appeal hearing was that the court simply wasn't interested. Lord Woolf wanted to know what we were talking about storage for. He pointed out that, in my case, the sperm was stored. Whether or not it should have been in the first place was immaterial. The court was trying to solve the problem as it presented itself at that moment in time, not go back to square one and solve a whole load of hypothetical situations. They didn't wish to waste their time. All my supporters must have breathed out in unison. It felt as though the room itself had just let out a huge sigh of relief. That was a whole section we simply didn't have to bother with.

Treatment abroad always appeared to me to be a less complex issue, involving only the will of the HFEA. There was no case of it being against the law to allow export. It was simply about whether the HFEA had the right to refuse in my particular circumstances. Any decision would not have any further implications. It could set no precedent. The situation was unique.

First, what we had called the domestic scrutiny issue. Was the HFEA's decision to refuse export one which a reasonable body of people could have come to? In deciding this, the court was obliged to apply the rigorous standards of judicial review appropriate in a case involving basic rights and freedoms. The HFEA were not allowed to fetter a discretion given to them by Parliament. If they never made any exceptions simply on the grounds that it would make an exception, they would never exercise their freedom to make individual decisions depending on different circumstances. There had to be some further justification and this had to be proportionate to their aims. This was one of the main differences to the first court case. In the lower court they had failed to give any reasons for their refusal. Now we had the four reasons given in November, after they had reconsidered the issue. We attacked all four. This was mostly covered by the HFEA's unwillingness to investigate the individual circumstances of our case, beyond the absence of written consent and the formalities required by domestic law. If we could have satisfied the requirements of UK law, the HFEA wouldn't have had to ask themselves if they would allow export in the first place, so this couldn't be a reason for denying it.

Within one of their reasons they had noted that I had no prior connection with any country to which I wished to export the sperm. This implied that maybe if we had been Belgian nationals or resident in Belgium, I could have had a direction to allow export. We put to the court that this was an irrelevant consideration, as well as being discriminatory both in purpose and effect. In law, you are not allowed to discriminate on the basis of nationality.

When I had first been given this reason by the HFEA and I had been asked for my response by the waiting journalists, I had really struggled to make my point succinctly. I had rambled on about no one having a problem with the fact that I had decided to use lawyers from London to argue my case, despite being from Nottinghamshire. If Nottinghamshire had some stupid law, I proposed that London wouldn't have a problem quashing it.

'Nottinghamshire is to London, what Europe, and therefore Brussels, is to London,' I reasoned.

Rather a long way around the houses to say what Lord Woolf managed to put in six words.

The HFEA's QC emphasised their point: 'Mrs Blood has no prior connection with Belgium.'

'Except that she is a European,' came Lord Woolf's response.

It was like light dawning. *Oh, yeah. That's what I was trying to say.*

The HFEA's final reason (well, actually it wasn't given as a reason – just something they'd borne in mind) – that my husband hadn't 'given any consideration, let alone consent, to the export of his sperm to another country' – we dismissed as being 'unrealistic and legalistic'. How could anyone possibly conclude that Stephen would have wanted me to have treatment but not if it meant going to a centre of medical excellence in Belgium, where the treatment was available? The court seemed to agree.

We'd just moved on to the European stuff when court ended for the day. I was feeling happy and encouraged by the judges' questions and responses. I therefore decided that perhaps I would make that trip to the theatre after all.

Following consultation with Gill and my parents, we decided to go and see *By Jeeves*. At least it meant that we weren't tempted to relive all the day's events by watching the reports of my case on TV that evening.

On the morning of day two, I was absolutely terrified. I'd had one day of happiness. I'd begun to see some hope of light at the end of the tunnel and I was frightened to death that, with the HFEA due to present their arguments today, my bubble was about to burst.

When I walked into court, I wondered what had happened. The whole place was full. Usually people sat quietly awaiting the arrival of the judges, but this day it seemed that everyone was talking at once and books were being paraded up and down the aisles, with their owners eagerly pointing out various references to the HFEA's legal team. *But this . . . But that . . . But the other . . .*

The HFEA's QC spoke to them, but didn't take the books. I

think he already had everything clear in his mind and didn't want to be distracted. I recognised the frustration on these people's faces and suddenly I understood. The judges had responded positively to some of the things my side had put forward and the HFEA's supporters were desperate to answer back. Now they knew how I had felt for the last year and ten months. When you believe in something with all your heart, you cannot understand how anyone could possibly disagree. The only explanation is that they have missed some vital point and to be denied the voice to explain is rather like having your hands tied behind your back and then being chastised for being unable to tie your shoelaces.

Proceedings began. My QC launched in at the point where we had left off the previous day. The European scrutiny issue was our strongest point. It began with the principle of the EC Treaty right to unhindered access to medical treatment throughout the member states of the Union. The only counter to this is where there is some overriding public policy argument against it. This was what the HFEA would try to prove.

At the lower court they had also relied on the fact that they were not hindering my right to go abroad to be inseminated. They were just preventing me from taking my husband's sperm with me. Obviously, in practical terms, this meant that I couldn't have the treatment I desired, even though I could still have treatment with the sperm of a stranger (treatment I could have had in Britain anyway). We aimed to show that preventing me from exporting my husband's sperm frustrated my aims in the same way as saying I could go abroad for medical services but couldn't take enough money with me to pay for it, or by denying me access to information regarding the availability of treatment overseas.

There was plenty of existing legal authority on both of these issues. In the latter case, at the European Court of Justice (ECJ) in Luxembourg, Ireland had lost its case against Open Door Counselling and Dublin Well Woman Clinic when the Government had tried to hinder girls seeking abortions in England by preventing the distribution of information and literature on the subject. This abortion issue was also a precedent which meant that I need have no prior connection with the country where I wished to be treated and that I could not be denied a medical operation that was legal abroad just because it was illegal in my own country.

What could probably have been prevented on the grounds of

public policy was something happening within Britain that was enforced on it by another country. For example, the HFEA relied on a case concerning the sale of lottery tickets in the UK at a time when such lotteries were unlawful in England. A prohibition on lottery operators from other member states advertising, marketing and selling lottery tickets within British territory was upheld by the ECJ. This was because it was 'a necessary part of the protection which that member state seeks to secure *within its territory*'. We added emphasis to the last three words in order to illustrate our point.

However, the equivalent of my case to this lottery ban would have been a restriction on British tourists buying lottery tickets whilst abroad in Germany, or in another member state where the provision of such services was lawful. Quite apart from the subject matter, it wasn't the same thing.

All this, of course, was my opinion and that of my legal team. The HFEA were about to start on theirs. That's when I just held my breath and prayed.

The judges also asked questions of the HFEA's QC and it was obvious that, just as they had understood and agreed with many of the points that we had made, they also agreed with many put forward by the HFEA. It was a long day. I spent most of it staring up at the three judges, hoping that they could read my mind whenever I wanted to barge in with one of my 'buts' in response to something David Pannick, the HFEA's QC, had said.

There were one or two high points. I remember at one stage being particularly frustrated at my inability to speak. David Pannick had been quoting from the Warnock Report, where it stated that they had 'grave misgivings' about posthumous insemination with a husband or partner's sperm. He was doing this to try and discern what the legislators had intended when they framed the Act in 1990. He made the very valid point that, at the time of my court case (which began in 1996), society probably held a much more liberal view than they had done six years earlier. We therefore could not take a view today and use that to judge what had been intended in 1990.

I really wanted to scream out: *the Warnock Report was written in 1984, six years before the Act. There is no difference between using that as a guide and using society's opinion today. You've just blown your own argument.*

In the absence of anyone else I could communicate with, I scribbled furiously to show my father and my solicitor, and fidgeted about on my seat, virtually hopping up and down.

Lord Woolf responded to David Pannick, 'Mmm, but wasn't the Warnock Report written in 1984?'

He didn't go on to make the rest of the connection. He didn't have to. I knew from that that he had taken on board the point I wanted to make. I breathed out and beamed from ear to ear. I wanted to show him that I was so glad he understood my point. I think he smiled back at me, but maybe it was because he was just so grateful that I'd stopped fidgeting.

There was a similar incident a little later. Lord Lester, my QC, knew I would be pleased and he wrote me a friendly little note. 'See, I told you Lord Woolf was a nice judge. Say now. He is, isn't he, whatever happens?'

I paused slightly before handing back my reply. It was committing myself somewhat to say that I believed I had had a fair crack at justice when I didn't know the outcome. It's not really something you can change your mind about later, if you lose. However, after brief consideration, I decided that I did believe it, so I scribbled 'yes' and sent the piece of paper back.

As the HFEA came towards the end of their submissions, it was a very tense time. I'd had another piece of paper handed to me from my QC. 'Watch the judges' body language now. This is when you'll win or lose.' I'm afraid I couldn't look after that. We'd had some highs. We'd had some lows. To be honest, I really didn't know which way it would go.

It was the end of day two. The HFEA still had to finish and then we got our chance for a brief response. Everyone was tired. Any lasting impressions had already been made.

Again, we decided to distract ourselves by going to the theatre. This time it was Alan Bennett's *Talking Heads*. The plays were very witty and I enjoyed the diversion. I know that Gill appreciated them, too. It was nice to see her laughing. It seemed a long time since I'd seen her face so illuminated. It was the glimmer of hope. During the days we were so busy trying to follow the legal arguments that we had no time to dwell on the sadness of Steph's death or the fear of losing the appeal. Going to the theatre stopped us from harbouring such thoughts at night, although it was, of course, impossible to forget completely.

At the interval, a member of the audience negotiated her way between the seats to wish me luck. I've no idea who she was, but it was a nice touch and I appreciated her kind wishes. I still felt I needed all the luck I could get.

The case finished at lunchtime on the third day. It had been another of those horrendous clock-watching exercises. David Pannick had talked for just long enough to put the pressure on to finish before lunch but not left quite the gap that might have been desired to fit our response within that period. I was concerned that Lord Lester should make all our points without it becoming tedious. Difficult, when everyone is anxious to finish.

The clock ticked round and we were heading for a late lunch. We just had one more reference to make. There was much scuffling whilst we rummaged among the papers to find it. The delay seemed a lifetime. If only they would call a break for lunch, then we could all talk, make sure we'd covered everything and find this stupid reference without the pressure of everyone's eyes bearing down on us.

Lord Woolf suggested that perhaps we should have a five-minute recess whilst everyone went to the toilet. Like most people in the court that morning, by that time I was desperate to go to the loo, but I was relieved in more ways than one.

There was an embarrassingly loud chorus of 'Phew' and then slight nervous giggling and chit chat, as temporarily the pressure was released. I queued for the toilet, we sorted ourselves out and filed back into court.

We were able to finish making our points and Lord Woolf concluded that, naturally, judgement would be deferred, but he promised that we wouldn't have too long to wait.

We left the Court of Appeal in a mood of wary optimism. It had definitely gone much better than the first hearing, but no one was willing to place any bets. My entire legal team, my family and I went for a meal just down the road from the court. It gave us the chance to dissect how it had gone. We chatted happily and joked about who would play the various characters when they made the film of my story. We had reason to hope I would win, but at the end of the day we simply didn't know. I'm not sure these things can bear too much scrutiny.

CHAPTER 15

Court of Appeal judgement

One week passed and then two. Why was there still no news of a forthcoming decision? To start off with, I had coped well with the wait. I kept myself busy and cheerful. I spring-cleaned the house (despite it being the middle of winter) and I threw myself into work. My biggest fear was winning, only for the HFEA to appeal.

Slowly, though, things became more difficult. My heart sank and my energy drained completely. The longer the wait became, the more I began to interpret it as bad news. Perhaps the judges couldn't agree, or maybe the longer they had thought about it, the more they had been convinced by the HFEA's argument, forgetting all the positive things they had said in the courtroom.

Melanie Phillips wrote a highly inaccurate and invasive article about myself and my late husband in *The Observer* on 26 January 1997. Amongst other details, she included falsely emotive and graphic descriptions of what my husband had endured on his deathbed, and said it was 'an appalling way to treat a dying person'. Stephen did die in agony, but not through anything that I or any doctor imposed. Anyone who has witnessed the ravages of meningitis will testify as to its horror. By the time his semen was taken, my beloved and beautiful husband was calm, stable and could feel nothing. The doctors had lodged evidence to that effect on my behalf. In a way it is sad, because I would like to think that Steph had felt me holding his hand.

Melanie Phillips believed that the court would rule in my favour, but she suggested that they should not. She warned the Master of the Rolls, Lord Woolf, against using his office 'to extend the law regardless of Parliament's decision'. Only a decision against my wishes, she argued, would uphold 'certainty and parliamentary authority', in addition to making 'a stand for the interests of the child'. But the law wasn't a 'certainty'. That's why I was given leave to go to the Court of Appeal in the first place and why we were now waiting for the clarification of a judgement. Of all the articles written against me, I found this one the most offensive. Whilst awaiting judgement (as at the lower court and whilst waiting for the HFEA to reconsider the export question), I had remained silent in the press. However, I could not let this incident pass without comment. It was clearly written with the aim of influencing the court and, although I didn't think the judges needed lessons in justice from either Melanie Phillips or myself, I felt obliged to correct the record. Lord Lester, my QC, contacted the editor of *The Observer* on my behalf and I was granted the right to reply.

The Observer, being a Sunday broadsheet, is only published once a week, so I had a few days to frame my reply. I suppose it kept me busy and focused for a while; although the clock still ticked as though a magnet were pulling its hands backwards.

The 5th of February 1997 was the day before what would have been Stephen's 32nd birthday. Three weeks had passed since the end of the appeal and still we had heard nothing. I occupied myself by going to buy some flowers for his grave. I had purchased a banner proclaiming 'Happy Birthday' the previous Saturday, and my intention was to fix it around his headstone. Cemeteries can be such sombre places; I thought Steph would appreciate me brightening it up somewhat.

I considered waiting and going up on his birthday, but the weather was fair and I couldn't guarantee what it would be like the following day. Also, I was feeling particularly low and I needed the solace. Accordingly, I walked up the long lines of graves until I reached Stephen's sundial.

I laid the flowers out on the ground and arranged them neatly in the two pots, muttering to myself, or to Steph, as I did so. Next, I wrapped the banner around the stone and fixed it in place with sticky tape.

The job done, I just stood back and prayed silently, 'Please don't let this go on any more. Please give the judges the wisdom to grant us justice soon and tell Steph I love him and I hope he has a good birthday.'

I opened my eyes, sensing someone's presence. It was a man walking towards me. He was closer than I had anticipated.

'Sorry, duck,' he ventured in a local accent, which reminded me of my husband. 'I just wanted to wish you luck.'

I thanked the stranger and started to leave. I had only gone a few paces when my handbag started ringing. Rather embarrassed at having left my mobile phone turned on in such a sacred place, I scrabbled around in the bottom of the bag in a desperate attempt to find and answer it quickly. It was Lord Lester, my QC. They'd just heard. Judgement was to be given in the morning – Steph's birthday. It had to be a good omen.

I called my parents in a bit of a flap. It didn't leave us long to get down there and organise a hotel. We couldn't risk travelling in the morning and arriving late. A few more phone calls to various members of the legal team and we had managed to confirm all the essential details I had forgotten to ask when I had first been told. We now knew the time of the judgement was 10 a.m. and that we had to attend a conference the hour before in Counsel's chambers. We tried to work out why we had been given hardly any warning by the judges. The prominent theory seemed to be that the judges hadn't wanted to give the press time to whip up a storm first. Another supposition was that they had only just finished writing the judgement and, being aware of their promise not to take too long, had wanted to let us know as soon as possible. Apparently, they didn't even normally give judgements on Thursdays, the day of the week on which Steph's birthday fell. My own theory was that God must have answered my prayer.

In a flurry of excitement, I called Stephen's parents. They couldn't make the trip at such short notice but were delighted that we would soon know the outcome. Like myself, Gill, Steph's mum, was convinced that it was good omen that it would be on Stephen's birthday. After being fairly insistent that I should wear my blue suit (Stephen's favourite colour), she said she felt sure that 'we were going to get it this time'.

I threw my belongings into a case and ignored the ringing telephones whilst I waited for my parents to arrive. It seemed the press had been informed, or more likely tipped off, by some court official, almost simultaneously with myself. They all wanted to know my arrangements. I don't think anyone believed me that I'd only just heard myself that the judgement was to be tomorrow.

My parents arrived and I piled everything into the car. I probably took far too many clothes, but I couldn't think what I needed. Lord Lester had invited us to the House of Lords that evening to hear a debate on the Human Rights Bill, which he had been trying to get through Parliament for some time. As we were going to be in London anyway for the evening, I thought it would be interesting to go. What do you need for an evening at the House of Lords, a morning in court and an unspecified number of TV and press interviews? Whatever was required, I was bound to have forgotten something.

We were soon on our way. We didn't have much time to check into the hotel and get changed before we had to be at the House of Lords. As we arrived, they were just having a vote on the previous issue so everyone was milling around in the lobby. I caught a glimpse of Baroness Warnock heading towards the cloakroom, so I flew across to tell her my news about the judgement being tomorrow. She asked where I wanted to have treatment if I won. I told her Belgium, on account of the clinic's excellent reputation and because it had been carefully considered by their Ethics Committee. She seemed happy for me. I must have radiated confidence for her to have asked such an optimistic question, but inside I was still extremely frightened.

The debate was stimulating and held my interest. It was pertinent to me because if the European Convention on Human Rights had been incorporated fully into English law, it just might have helped my case. As it was, it was something which could directly assist only if I took my case as far as Europe. This seemed most unfair. Most abuses of human rights are, by their nature, cases of individuals versus the state, and the state can generally run an oppressed person out of energy and money. The longer they can string a case out, forcing the individual through as many courts as possible, the more likely they are to win by default. This is not justice. It's tyranny.

One of the main arguments against introducing a Human Rights Bill seemed to be that, with Europe as a safety net, we didn't need one. Also, it would erode British sovereignty. This seemed incredibly arrogant to me. The United States, plus virtually every country in Europe, barring Britain, already assured human rights by statute. The saying 'free born Englishman' was absolute rubbish. What it really meant was free to do anything unless there is a piece of legislation which says otherwise, or if the authorities choose to introduce one at any point during your lifetime. As freedom is a matter of trust, I did not see where the problem lay in issuing a guarantee.

Human rights law was, and still is, something with which many people disagree. Campaigners, most notably Lord Lester, had been trying to introduce the Bill for around the last 30 years, irrespective of which government had been in power at the time. This final attempt looked like it might succeed, particularly if Labour came to power after the next general election. A limitation clause had been added which, roughly interpreted, meant that, when introducing new laws, the Government would be able to exclude any part of the Human Rights Bill at any time, so long as they stated that they intended doing so at the time the statute was framed. At least this would help avoid mistakes such as those I believed they had made when they drew up the 1990 Human Fertilisation and Embryology Act. They didn't realise they would infringe any basic human rights in a situation such as mine, because, quite simply (as per the evidence of Baroness Warnock), a situation such as mine had never occurred to them.

Lord Alderdice flew in especially for the debate from Northern Ireland. He gave a particularly moving speech, reminding everyone that Northern Ireland is also part of the British Isles. Given the infringements that can occur over there, after what he said, I would have thought it hard for anyone from England, Wales or Scotland to feel they had any right to offer any opposition at all.

Lord Woolf also spoke at the debate. He was seated on the cross-party benches, which were only a few feet from where I was sitting. It was strange to think that in the morning I would be sitting in his court. What's more, at that very moment, he already knew my fate. I wondered if he noticed me. His face wasn't giving away any clues.

The following morning, we all met at Counsel's chambers. Any second, I would know the result. As I walked in, I almost bumped into Ruth Deech of the HFEA. She was standing just behind the door in the waiting room. She was there to see her barristers for the same reason as I was there to see mine. I wondered if she already knew. I couldn't tell anything by her face, save the surprise of having her space accidentally invaded by an anxious 30 year old. It was nerve-shattering.

We said hello to one another and she left the room moments later. She looked like she was heading into a meeting rather than just leaving, so I concluded that perhaps she hadn't known the outcome at that moment after all. My solicitor arrived and then we went into our own meeting. I was accompanied by my parents.

Copies of the judgement were clutched in Lord Lester's hand. We all drew in our breath and held it until someone spoke.

'Well, it's good, but you're not quite there yet.'

'What do you mean?'

Quickly, my legal team explained. It was a unanimous decision. The court's ruling meant that I couldn't be treated in England, but they had thrown the decision on export back to the HFEA. They had clarified two points of law which they felt were important for members of the HFEA to take into account. First, that I did have a right to export the sperm under EC law, and second, that my situation could never recur. They were looking at a one-off situation which could set no precedent. The reason for this was that it had now been confirmed that, from now on, to commence storage of sperm in Britain without written consent from the donor was illegal, although in my case no one could be blamed, as it was a previously unexplored area of law.

Basically, this left the HFEA with little alternative but to agree to my wishes on exportation. They could only refuse if they could demonstrate that there was a public policy reason why Diane Blood, as one sole individual, with 90 per cent of the population behind her and with what both courts had described as 'compelling' evidence as to her husband's wishes, should not be allowed to export his sperm. In particular, the Court of Appeal indicated that it probably would be unlawful to continue to refuse to make a direction to allow export. The judgement made clear that the refusal of a direction infringed my legal rights, and stated that it was 'unlikely' that any of the concerns identified by the Authority could be a lawful justification for that infringement.

'You have won the appeal and it means you will get what you want. It's just that you have to be patient for a little while longer,' the team assured me.

On an intellectual level, I agreed. There couldn't be any possible public policy that could stand against me, as an isolated case. What happened in my little family was hardly likely to rock the foundations of society.

I read the judgement, but I still wasn't totally convinced. I believed I must have some supporters within the HFEA but was sure the Authority would still refuse export. In answer to this, my legal team explained that it was very important to get leave to go back to the same court if they did refuse, otherwise we'd have to start all over again, explaining everything to a new set of judges.

We were running out of time. We still had to walk across to the court, make it through the barrage of cameras and be seated before ten. Quickly, we left the chambers and continued talking en route. As we had won the appeal, we could also ask for our costs, although this would probably be disputed by the HFEA. As a very rough guess, the claimable cost of the court action for both sides together would be somewhere in the region of £150,000. The HFEA would argue that I should only receive a portion of my costs, as we had argued three points and I had only been proved right on the export issue. We would disagree. If they'd agreed to export in the first place, I'd have been happy and we'd never have been in court.

We stopped talking when we came within earshot of the reporters. Microphones were thrust in front of us from people wanting to know if I had won the right to try for Stephen's baby. I told them that they would have to wait and see. Perhaps what I should have said is, *I'm not quite sure. I'll have to wait and see.*

The judges filed into court almost simultaneously with ourselves and the media entourage. The court was organised. It had prepared a typed summary of the judgement on single A4 sheets to hand out to the journalists. My solicitor joked about the judges distributing their own press release.

The sheets were handed out and then Lord Woolf basically read out what was written on the summary, adding that the court regretted if their decision should prolong my agonising predicament any longer. The HFEA gave a date when they would reconsider export at the end of the month. I was grateful. At least I wasn't going to be left in limbo again, not knowing when a decision was to be made.

Rapidly, we moved on to other business. Lord Lester asked for leave to apply and return to the same court should the HFEA still refuse export. This was granted easily, although the judges looked a bit baffled as to why we thought we might need it. It was going well.

Now on to costs. The HFEA opposed our application for costs, either wholly or partially, on the grounds that they had been proved right on domestic law. Lord Lester stood up and disagreed, but then he made a mistake, saying that we weren't asking for costs for the initial leave hearing. Michael Fordham, his junior, prodded him frantically in the back to correct him on this. The judges didn't notice. They disappeared into a little huddle to discuss it amongst themselves. It took all of two seconds. They cannot have had the chance to say much. Lord Lester barged back in before Lord Woolf opened his mouth to give the decision.

'My Lord . . .' He began to explain his mistake, saying that he hadn't meant to exclude the leave hearing.

Lord Woolf interrupted. They were going to award all my costs anyway, irrespective of what Lord Lester had said.

I was absolutely over the moon. I knew some expenses would be disallowed, but I had been given so much. The judges were so positive, I was sure the HFEA would grant export and now I wouldn't be left financially impaired to the extent that I would struggle to provide for our baby. What was more, it gradually dawned on me that I had been given the best judgement I could possibly have had. Quite apart from the fact that it was unanimous, in any event, it was the one decision that the HFEA could not appeal against. *Yes! Happy birthday, Steph!*

When we came out of court, Ruth Deech read a statement to the waiting journalists. She said that it was 'a judgement of Solomon, which everyone can be very pleased about. This is a unique case that will not open the floodgates.'

Only later in an interview for the *New Statesman* on 10 April did she appear to change this, saying mine was 'not a one-off case' and that she thought, 'most of the Authority thinks what happened was quite wrong. We're not happy that – sperm having been wrongly taken and the doctor having arguably assaulted the patient – all that should be cured by a trip to Brussels.' I sensed that Ruth Deech's statement on leaving court had probably been written by the HFEA's lawyers, but at the time I had no reason to suspect that it didn't accurately reflect her views.

I agreed with Ruth Deech that it was 'a judgement of Solomon' and in my own words I described it as 'a victory for common sense and for justice'.

Coming out of court this time was a bit of a free-for-all. Joshua Rozenberg of the BBC apologised that he hadn't managed to organise the mob into any semblance of order. Ruth Deech had left the court first, so she had been surrounded by the reporters. When our party then tried to leave, we were met at the door by runners who explained the situation outside and asked us to wait until the HFEA had said their piece and gone. We couldn't have got past them anyway. There was such a crowd.

The media messengers avoided the need for us to keep peering outside. They chased backwards and forwards with updates until they eventually gave us the all-clear.

'You can come now. It's your turn. We'll try to hold them back. Are you ready?'

I held my breath and my solicitor, my family and I were ushered to the centre of the pack. The people closest to us tried to form a barrier to stop us from being crushed, but it was difficult. They were being trampled on from behind and found it impossible to maintain a steady footing. The sea of reporters swayed backwards and forwards, with us enclosed in their midst: a few fragile bodies set adrift on a rather unstable dinghy.

The rest of the day was filled with champagne and non-stop interviews. We held a press conference (where I decided to photograph the photographers and journalists for a change). It went on for what must have been a good couple of hours because when I'd finished answering the general questions, they all kept trying to grab me for a quick 'exclusive' aside. I thought that one journalist, Mary Riddell, who at that time was writing for the *Daily Mirror*, had had more than her fair share of time. However, when I read her article in the paper, I forgave her entirely. If I criticised Melanie Phillips for her piece before the judgement, then equally I must praise Mary Riddell for writing the only article throughout my case which I could single out as being not only entirely accurate but also incredibly perceptive. I was amazed how she had gleaned so much insight into my character, let alone factual information, in the middle of a crowded press conference from someone who, at that moment, was rather tired and not exactly the most willing interviewee.

Court of Appeal judgement

It wasn't over. Demands were still being made on my time. The press deadline had passed, but there was work to be done for TV and radio. We travelled from studio to studio. I couldn't ignore it because the HFEA were also doing the rounds. The controversy was far from over. The media interpreted the judgement as the court handing the HFEA a 'fig leaf', or a way of giving in without losing face. They had effectively been told to go away and come up with the right answer next time. I think this annoyed them somewhat. Ruth Deech gave interviews saying that they might well still refuse export.

I found it all deeply distressing, but I could hardly be pessimistic. The facts just didn't stand up. There could be no earthly reason for them to refuse.

CHAPTER 16

The HFEA reconsider again

Over the next few weeks, we were kept busy preparing for the HFEA's meeting on 27 February – another significant date, sandwiched between the date my husband fell ill with meningitis two years earlier and the date he had suffered the cardiac arrest. I wasn't quite sure whether to take that as a good or bad omen.

Just because the court case was over didn't mean that there wasn't legal work to be done. David Pannick QC and Dinah Rose, the HFEA's barristers, had written their joint opinion for the meeting the day after the judgement. It was forwarded to us on 13 February. It was reasonably succinct and did point out to HFEA members that it was 'unlikely that the reasons previously given by the Authority could, in the exceptional circumstances of this case, satisfy the test of necessity and proportionality'. It went on to clarify this further, saying that:

> The Court of Appeal had explained that the concepts of 'necessity' and 'proportionality' mean that the Authority should only refuse Mrs Blood permission to export the sperm if satisfied that this is justified by some imperative requirement in the public interest, that the decision is suitable for securing the attainment of the objects which the Authority is pursuing, and the Authority is not going beyond what is necessary to attain the objective.

All rather legalistic stuff, but I was pleased that, for once, the HFEA's lawyers were basically telling them the same as mine were telling me.

Our side then had to prepare our own submissions. Both these and those prepared by the HFEA's Counsel would then be presented to the Authority members for them to consider in advance of their meeting. We did try to keep our observations short and sweet, but, as usual, there was so much we wanted to say and reiterate. It would have been easier if we could just have been there to answer questions, but we were trying to second guess all the perceived problems that anyone could possibly come up with. Whenever we submitted any arguments or evidence, I was always worried in case we'd missed anything important. It's rather like packing your suitcase to go on holiday. When you get to the airport, you're always anxious in case you've forgotten to include something.

The media were still chasing me for interviews and offering to pay large sums of money for the privilege. Apart from the immediate aftermath of the judgement, as at previous times when my fate had been in the balance, I refused.

Some people had criticised me throughout for holding conferences and getting involved with the media at all. Some criticised me for my periods of silence. I don't really know what I was supposed to do. Perhaps the HFEA's supporters saw the Authority as being unbiased, and therefore believed that only they should be allowed a voice. After all, it was their side who had blown the story open in the first place with their statement to the BBC. Perhaps I should have appeared secretive and afraid whilst the media camped outside my home and hassled my friends and family, frustrated at being able to glean nothing from me. I really do not know. One thing I do know is that, at times, the decisions I had to make regarding the media were agonising. They were not motivated by money. (I never accepted any deals.) Neither were they motivated by the desire to be famous. At times I sat cowering by the phone, dreading the sound of its ring, not knowing what to say or who would be on the other end of the line. A friend of mine, on witnessing the distress this could cause, wondered why I did not change my phone number and go ex-directory.

Escape is not so easy. You would have to cut yourself off entirely from society: live nowhere, work nowhere and talk to no one. At times throughout my ordeal, in an attempt to avoid attention, I headed towards this total isolation and discovered it was unbearable.

For my part, if I had changed my home number, so long as I wanted to earn money, I would still have needed a work and mobile phone number. Working, as I do, in PR and advertising, the media have to have those phone numbers. It is the business I had always worked in. I did not have a secretary to block my calls or a bodyguard to protect me from media attention when I ventured onto the street. I was just doing the best I knew how with a very difficult set of circumstances. At the end of the day, it was and still is me who has to deal with the consequences of my actions or, equally, my inaction. I honestly believe that anyone who has never been in my position has no right to judge.

Another difficult call, not relating directly to the press but regarding publicity in a roundabout sort of way, came during that month of February. I was invited to speak to sixth-form pupils at Westminster School in London on the day before the HFEA's meeting. If I accepted, I would have to speak to a large group for around 20 minutes, answer their questions and then I would be invited to lunch with selected students from their midst. I was a bit nervous about shouting my cause before the HFEA's meeting, but the lecturer assured me that no journalists would be present and, in any case, with only one day to go to the meeting, it would be a bit late to have any effect anyway. I agreed that perhaps I was being a little paranoid. I couldn't go through the rest of my life fearing that every time I opened my mouth, even in private, someone somewhere was going to report it. Besides, I thought it would be great to see the school. It costs a great deal of money to send children there and I was curious to compare it to the comprehensive which I had attended.

I did, however, have one other rather large and selfish hang-up – the age of my audience. To put it bluntly, I didn't think they'd be very sympathetic. I thought they couldn't possibly project themselves into the mind of a 30-year-old woman and imagine what it was like to lose someone you had loved for 12 years, let alone understand the biological desire to be a mother. This factor almost led to my refusal, but then I realised how incredibly narrow-minded that made me.

I agreed to go to Westminster School and wrote my speech on

prejudice. It took me the best part of a weekend to complete, so I was glad they seemed to appreciate it. Until I actually timed it, I had no idea just how many words you need to say to fill 20 minutes. I was very nervous, but the students were great. I told them how I had nearly pre-judged their reaction to me and used this to explain how unfairly I felt I had been treated when the HFEA had first made up their mind on the export issue before the very first court case and before they knew any facts or any evidence had ever been submitted. I felt my position had been prejudiced by their own opinion of my motivation. The same could be said of the BMA's Dr Stuart Horner, who judged me on what he had read in the newspapers. None of these people had ever met me, yet they judged me in the same way as I had judged these teenagers before I had met them. I concluded by saying that I ought to have known better.

After lunch, I got a guided tour of the school and a book as a memento of my visit. Everyone was very kind to me and they all wished me luck for the following day. It was all rather pleasant and it helped keep my mind occupied. I really had to be in London for the HFEA's decision anyway, just in case they came up with the wrong answer and we had to rush back into court. Had I been left sitting in a hotel room to contemplate my potential fate, I would have probably driven myself crazy. More banal distractions, such as TV, radio or books, simply didn't work. I tried reading the new book I had been given in order to help me go to sleep that night, but it was a total waste of time. I could neither read nor sleep.

Next morning I went to see Michael Fordham, my barrister. I wanted to take him a cartoon about my case. My solicitor had obtained the artwork from the newspaper who'd published it and I'd had some copies framed. Then I had to go for a meeting which my dad had arranged for us at the solicitors. It was nothing to do with the pending HFEA decision. It was to meet the cost clerk and try and get the process underway for recovering my legal fees.

The cost clerk told me what I could and couldn't claim for. Media-related expenses, such as the media training and conference rooms, obviously wouldn't be covered and neither would travel or hotel bills. They could maybe try to recoup the cost of those necessitated only by my own attendance at the court hearings but not those for meetings with lawyers or barristers or any costs in relation to my family who I had asked to accompany me. He explained that you only usually manage to recoup around 60 per cent of your costs. Thank goodness for the Stephen Blood Baby Appeal, which might help cover some of the rest. As I was from Nottinghamshire, for example, I was advised that I would only be allowed the expense of provincial lawyers. It was my choice that I had gone to London. But I'd tried the barrister from Nottingham and hadn't thought his advice was comprehensive enough. I would have found it all the more distressing that so many things were disallowed if I had been able to concentrate, but my mind was elsewhere and, at the end of the day, it was the HFEA's decision that was all-important, not the money.

Thankfully, I don't really think my solicitors had really planned to achieve a great deal from my meeting with the cost clerk anyway. In the end, I think we claimed somewhere in the region of £85,000, but we didn't do any sums until much later. At the time, I think it was more of a conspiracy between the solicitors and my dad to get me out of the hotel and prevent me from dwelling on the HFEA's meeting, which by then would have already been under way.

We had no idea what time the meeting would end or when I could expect to hear the verdict. Once again, our only clue came from the media. The HFEA had arranged a press conference for 4.30 p.m., so, logically, they would have to tell me before that. After consultation with the hotel manager, we told the press that I would be sitting in my hotel bar waiting to hear from 2 p.m. If they wanted to come and wait with me, then they were quite welcome.

They were already waiting for me in the lobby by the time I returned from the solicitor's a few minutes before two. I walked through the door with my dad, everyone stood up and the place suddenly lit up like a Christmas tree. Cameras were rolling and all lights were focused on me. I held my hand up in front of my eyes, unable to focus on a great deal. I felt like a startled rabbit. The glare was blinding.

'Hey, what's the rush? I'm not going anywhere,' I pleaded. 'Will you please give me a chance to go up to my room and freshen up before you start filming?'

Lights and cameras were instantaneously turned off. They checked that there weren't any escape routes, watched me go into the lift and said that they would be waiting and start filming as soon as I came down again. I agreed, pressed the number for my floor and the lift doors slowly drew across the scene. Now I could breathe out again. The shock of suddenly being in the spotlight had quite taken me aback.

My father and I both made our way to our respective rooms and reported to my mother on the throng waiting for us downstairs. We all got ready and then met up prior to going back down in the lift. It was rather intimidating watching the floor numbers count themselves back down. Five . . . four . . . three . . . two . . . one . . . and . . . lights . . doors open . . . you're on.

The questions started almost immediately. They all wanted to know what the HFEA had decided. So did I, but I thought we'd made it plain that at two o'clock I wouldn't know. Maybe they thought I'd tricked them, or perhaps that I had some special power that enabled me to project myself into the HFEA meeting and read their minds.

The hotel had given us the use of a room just off from the bar. I thought we'd better file in there for a while, just to clear up the confusion. The room was adequate but a little cramped, due to a huge, oval mahogany table, which took up virtually all the floor space. Most press conferences have a long head table where the interviewees are seated. The press then jostle for position on rows in front of it. With everyone standing or sitting around the perimeter of the table, this conference felt more like a meeting at King Arthur's court.

'I don't know the decision yet . . . No, I don't know which way it will go. What do you think? No, I don't know when I'll hear . . . You told me the HFEA have a press conference at 4.30 p.m. When do you think I'll get to know?' I wasn't answering questions so much as holding a two-way discussion.

When the press were satisfied that I wasn't hiding anything and didn't have any secret knowledge, we all retired to the bar. And there we waited for what seemed like an eternity. I passed the time by chatting with photographers and reporters. Obviously I was a bit wary about what I said, but these were respected as private conversations. They were not reported.

Most of the journalists were also supposed to be at the HFEA's conference at 4.30. If I didn't get the decision until late, they didn't know how they were supposed to cover both. Content that an afternoon chatting in a bar was a better than average day's work and that they were going to hear the decision from me anyway, most decided to stay put rather than chase around London trying to do the impossible.

Many of the photographers had been at the HFEA's offices in the morning. They had wanted to photograph members as they went into the meeting. They had waited for ages but seen no one, so it was a bit of a mystery as to how members had sneaked past unnoticed. It was February and the photographers had got rather cold hanging around, so they weren't that impressed that it had all been in vain.

The TV reporters had another tale to relate. They tried to persuade me to commit to doing evening interviews in their studios. I was told that the HFEA had briefed several of their members so they were equipped to go out and be interviewed in a variety of different places at once. This would avoid Ruth Deech trying to do it all. I wondered how I could split myself into pieces. I had to do it all myself, although I do admit I had the assistance of Stephen's former work colleagues from the Stephen Blood Baby Appeal, who'd always done a brilliant job of scheduling. One reporter from Central TV had followed me around after one of the judgements until she made sure I hit her slot. She had been feeding me orange juice and had joined me in a rather valiant run across a pitch-black area of grass to make it to some shed in time to be interviewed for BBC *World News*. She joked that she had never seen anyone perform so many interviews in such a short space of time. Wherever I popped up, though, the opposition always seemed to be there as well, so the HFEA must also qualify for the record.

This time, if the decision went my way, I didn't really care who was interviewed where. It wouldn't make any difference any more. They could say what they liked. I told the TV reporters that I would have to see what the decision was before I would commit to any interviews afterwards.

For me, the worst news of the day was Dolly the sheep. Scientists had managed to clone a sheep and had just released the story that afternoon. For some bizarre reason that I will never understand, this somehow managed to get linked to me. I think the 'logic' ran something along the lines of that people like myself, who had lost their spouses, would wish to clone their deceased loved ones in order to somehow bring them back to life. This again goes back to what I see as one of the basic misunderstandings about my wishes.

My desire to have my husband's baby was not triggered by his death. It preceded his death. I would be no more likely to want a clone of him now than I would have if he'd been alive. The idea is stupid.

As for Dolly, I'm sure she was a very nice sheep. I had nothing against her personally or the basic technology that brought about her existence. Perhaps it could help lead to a cure for cancer or some of our more devastating diseases. Actually proceeding to full human cloning is another issue. It is currently fraught with difficulties and possibly devastating consequences. I think it is unsafe to experiment with this technology on human offspring and I do not believe that position is likely to change for an extremely long time. If it was safe, then I don't particularly think that producing the odd clone would irreparably damage the fabric of human society. After all, identical twins share not only the same DNA (like clones) but also the same womb and upbringing, so they would be even more alike. It's just that, to be honest, I can't see why anyone would think that cloning was a desirable method of reproduction. To me, the diversity and randomness of human life is what makes it so amazingly wonderful. I wanted to combine my genetic material with that of the man I loved, and I do not understand why I was linked to technology over which I had no control and in which I had no direct interest.

Neither, to be honest, do I understand the media's seemingly irrelevant preoccupation with commenting on hypothetical situations. They spend so much time debating situations that seem so unlikely to happen. I think I agree with the courts on this one. We have enough real conundrums to solve without getting into the realms of 'What if?'

Throughout my court case, the media repeatedly asked if I would agree with a situation where a man wanted to use his deceased wife's eggs in the same way as I wanted to use my husband's sperm. Obviously, this would mean the need for a surrogate mother, which gives an added dimension to the problem. I pointed out the practicalities of her needing to die at the moment of ovulation and that, unless she was in the middle of fertility treatment anyway (and therefore would have had the chance to sign the relevant consent form, making it legal), she would probably only have one egg, giving virtually zero chance of fertilisation. Perhaps I should simply have pointed out that at that time, we didn't even know how to freeze eggs anyway, so the question was redundant. With a woman, you would have had to have taken the rather uncertain alternative of freezing ovarian tissue, which, incidentally, would also have been perfectly legal. I think that everyone imagines science to be far more advanced than it is.

There certainly seems to be a rather false notion that once you have produced an embryo, a successful pregnancy is bound to occur. This is not true. The majority of IVF attempts fail after the implantation of an embryo. Many natural pregnancies also fail at this stage. I think we all had it drummed into us at school that the first time we even thought about sex, the girl was going to end up pregnant. It might have been more honest (and less likely to make the one in five who subsequently discover they have fertility problems feel like a failure) if someone had pointed out that actually it's technically so difficult to conceive that it's a miracle it ever happens at all.

If I won the right to export my husband's sperm, I knew that there were no guarantees that it would result in a baby. With an average success rate of around 20 per cent per cycle of treatment, I thought the odds were pretty reasonable, but I was only fighting for the right to try. The rest was up to God.

Right now, though, it was in the hands of the HFEA, and the couple of hours spent waiting for their answer seemed like a lifetime. We were all sitting looking at our watches, thinking that it couldn't take much longer, and every time a mobile phone rang, the whole room jumped up in anticipation. Was this the call to say they were ready to fax the verdict?

At one point, I was handed a piece of paper. I wondered what had happened, as suddenly I was surrounded and the camera lights beamed down on me. I opened the paper and read its contents. It was a message from the BBC asking if my solicitor would appear on *Newsnight* that evening. The lights were turned off and everyone sat down again, groaning with disappointment.

When the call did eventually arrive, I almost missed it. It was 4.15 p.m. Richard Stein, my solicitor, had been talking to his secretary for a while. The decision had been faxed to Leigh, Day and they were sending it straight on to us. She briefly imparted the contents to Richard. As realisation dawned, a general hush fell over the assembly of reporters. Any second now, I would know.

He ended the conversation and walked over, beaming.

'Have I got it?' I screeched in a high-pitched, nervous voice.

He nodded. 'It is being faxed to us now. There are conditions, but it looks OK.'

I was hemmed in on a settee in the corner of the bar. All cameras focused on me, expecting some grand speech, but I hadn't thought what to say. I just couldn't believe it was true, that finally it was all over.

The reporters wanted to crack the champagne, but I wouldn't let them. 'Not yet. We need to read the conditions.'

We filed back into the room with the large oval table whilst awaiting the arrival of the fax. My family, solicitor and I were seated farthest from the door. Several curly, flimsy bits of paper were handed down the room to us. It was the HFEA's export directions for the sperm. Eagerly we pored over the conditions in full view of the world's media. There were loads of them and it all looked a bit technical, but neither Richard nor I could find anything which was cause to stop the celebration. The HFEA confirmed at their press conference that it contained nothing which should worry me, and their comments were fed directly back to me by the journalists who were with me. They wanted me to stop worrying and get on with the party before they missed their deadlines.

Finally, I spoke. 'All right, it seems OK. Let's get that champagne.'

So that was it. We went outside so I could shake the bottle and spray it over the waiting photographers. A couple of waiters from the hotel followed us outside with a silver tray and glasses, but I'm afraid all decorum went totally to the wind and I slurped straight from the bottle.

Why should I care any more? 'No, that's it. No more interviews. No more visits to TV studios. If you want to film me, you'll have to do it here.'

Satellite dishes were rapidly erected and we all stood freezing to death on various street corners within walking distance from the hotel. My entire legal team, Jane Atkinson (who'd helped with PR advice at various times) and almost everyone else who'd been involved all came down to see me. It was so wonderful to be happy. I couldn't remember the last time I did not have some huge shadow hanging over me. Now it was all-clear. I finally had my life back.

Michael Fordham, my barrister, waved frantically from across the road. He was beaming from ear to ear. He shouted his congratulations and motioned that he was going into the hotel to wait. I wanted to go inside, get warm and join my family and friends, but I just had one final interview to do for ITN. We moved to another street corner, where they were already set up and ready to roll.

'Your camera's facing the wrong way,' I joked.

There was a pub directly in front of me. Its sign, depicting a rather romantic-looking ship, overhung the pavement, silhouetted beautifully against the crisp February skies.

The crew looked rather puzzled at my comment.

'Look,' I pointed. 'The Victory.'

It was finally beginning to sink in.

With the interviews over, I retired back to the hotel for a celebratory meal with my lawyers, family and friends. Steph's family back home in Worksop knew of the decision because I had told them to watch the television. The news would be released the instant I knew and they would hear it from the media before I would have the chance to tell them in person. When we sat down for our meal, it was the first opportunity I had to ring them. Everyone was jubilant; Steph would have been thrilled.

My life was my own once again. I could now try to plan and go through my medical treatment without everyone knowing my every move. Neither I nor the hospital in Belgium would want the world's media following me there. I am far from alone in having to go through fertility treatment in order to try for the family I desired, and that particular journey is one which many can and have told. For me, I suspected it would be no different than it was for them. We would all desperately want to succeed and we would all be devastated in the face of failure. Of course, I didn't have the emotional support of a husband there beside me, but I could still take strength from his inspiration and dreams. Although the moment of medical conception is no great mystery and I am grateful and was indeed encouraged by others who have told of their experience, I had no intention of sharing with the world a blow-by-blow account of my particular treatment. In medical terms, there would be nothing unique about it, and I thought it was important to keep my life as stress-free and private as possible in order to maximise my chances of success.

CHAPTER 17

The start of the rest of my life

I think that everyone expected me to announce a pregnancy within a couple of months, but exporting the sperm, let alone arranging my treatment, took ages to organise. A clinic in Italy kindly offered to treat me free of charge, but my export directions specified the clinic that I had identified in Belgium and they did have an excellent reputation (one of the best, if not *the* best, in the world), so I decided to stick with them. If I had wanted to go to a different clinic, I would have had to go back to the HFEA and start again.

First, Professor Cooke was out of the country at a medical conference and then everyone thought that we should wait until the fuss died down. I went on a couple of short holidays with my friend Helen, who I had known since our schooldays. We went to Rome in May and then we tried to enjoy a few days in the Lake District in autumn, but the break was disrupted by the publication of the 'Consent and the Law' consultation document and questionnaire by Professor Sheila McLean on 24 September 1997. This was the review of the current provisions in the Human Fertilisation and Embryology Act 1990 that had been announced by Baroness Cumberlege at the end of the second reading of Lord Winston's Private Member's Bill.

Members of the public still had the opportunity to respond by answering questions that it posed, but it didn't look as though the report's final conclusions on posthumous conception were going to be particularly favourable, especially where there was no written consent. Also, this document's portrayal of the Court of Appeal judgement in my case seemed distorted and differed entirely from my own understanding. It claimed that the HFEA could still have refused me permission to export my husband's sperm and that, if they had done so, I would have been left with no legal remedy on the grounds that they were defending a public policy. Yet the judges had indicated this would be 'unlikely' and the HFEA's own lawyers had agreed. In an interview for the *New Statesman* on 10 April 1997, Ruth Deech said, 'But we were advised we would lose if we said no again. We were told by our lawyers we had to stop.' I was getting very frustrated at outside commentators playing judge. I wanted to set the record straight and the media wanted my comments.

I tried not to get too stressed by it. I no longer needed the law to be changed in order to be allowed to try for Steph's child, but the situation was difficult because I was not forewarned that the document was about to be released and I was therefore unprepared. My parents were not easy to contact, as they were on a boating holiday on the Shannon in Ireland. I remember making a frantic phone call to Lord Winston, asking him what to say, as I had no one else around who knew enough detail to give me an informed opinion. Lord Winston wondered why I should still care what the report said and wisely recommended that I should concentrate on enjoying my holiday. There was no need for me to become involved, as most of it could no longer affect me.

Still, I did care and, in due course, I responded to the Department of Health. The only question that was still relevant to me asked if the law should be amended to secure status and succession rights of children conceived after the death of a parent. This would be difficult, as it might make estates virtually impossible to wind up. I suggested that they should allow the father's name on the birth certificate, without necessarily affecting the inheritance issue.

Meanwhile, the fuss showed no signs of abating, but it was not so intense. Actually, I think that some people thought that, with no obstacles in my way and time to reflect, I might change my mind and decide not to try for my late husband's child after all.

When no news had materialised after almost 14 months, a family friend actually thought they should mention that they totally understood: 'What was important was that you won the right to make up your own mind. It doesn't matter if you decided not to go ahead in the end.'

I really wanted to point out that, whilst I appreciated the sentiment behind what they were saying, I wouldn't have risked everything that my husband and I had ever worked for if I was in any danger of ever changing my mind. As it was, I didn't reply. It was a bit awkward because I had promised my Belgian clinic that, given that they couldn't discuss my treatment due to medical confidentiality, I wouldn't discuss it either. More than anyone, I understand how difficult it is when someone else talks about something you are involved in whilst you must remain silent. I still will not discuss my treatment in detail for the same reason, but, in any case, at the time the press still regularly called my family and probably our friends to find out if there was any news. I didn't want anything I said to be innocently reported back to a newspaper. Only I knew of the hope I carried inside.

I was sitting on the bench in my front garden at home in Worksop, enjoying the sunny, spring Saturday morning of 26 April 1998, when suddenly an invigorating tingling sensation swelled in my breasts. Could this be the beginning of a new life? I dared not get too excited, but I was absolutely gutted when the following day it had disappeared. I prodded and poked in the hope that I could make the feeling return, but there was absolutely nothing. Dead as a dodo.

I had to wait until Wednesday (almost two weeks after my treatment in Belgium) for the pregnancy test at a local fertility clinic, which I had asked to monitor my hormones, before I reported the results to Belgium.

Paula, the nurse, asked if I had any inkling which way it would go.

'No.' I told her how my hopes had been raised, only to be dashed again.

'Well, we'll soon know one way or the other,' she assured me.

She was wrong. The pregnancy test proved positive, but only just. My HCG (human chorionic ganadotrophin) level was 25. We were looking for at least a 50. This could mean one of two things. Either the pregnancy was taking a while to establish itself and hadn't really got going yet, or a pregnancy had occurred and then terminated almost immediately. The odds were around 50/50 either way. I feared it was the latter. We would have to test again in three days' time.

HCG is a hormone which multiplies rapidly when you are pregnant, almost doubling every day. If it was good news, the levels would have risen dramatically. Bad news and it would probably have decreased.

On Saturday, my HCG was 43. There was still some hope but not a great deal. Even given the low start, it should have been at least 200.

We tried again the following Wednesday. The level was 107. It was still creeping up but not going as it should. That was when I was given the devastating news. The nurses felt it only fair to warn me that my body wasn't reacting as though it was a normal pregnancy. The most likely explanation was that there was a pregnancy, but it was ectopic, growing in my fallopian tubes or somewhere outside my womb. Assuming this to be the case, the baby could not be saved and I would have to have an operation in order to prevent my own life being put at risk.

I was totally bewildered. How could this happen? An ectopic pregnancy is a pretty unlikely event in the first place, but, if anything, it is actually less likely to occur with an assisted pregnancy than it is with a natural one. When I was three years old, I had watched my mother almost die from a pulmonary embolism following an emergency operation for an ectopic pregnancy. It was the last thing I wanted to hear. I was absolutely petrified. I was sitting on my own in a fertility clinic with no one there to comfort me. I was in such a state, I didn't know how I'd manage to drive home.

The nurses tried to assure me that, because I needed artificial assistance to become pregnant, I didn't need my fallopian tubes anyway. This was beside the point. I really missed having Steph's support. My emotions were in total turmoil. I'd gone from praying that I was pregnant to knowing that the best hope was that I wasn't. I wept for our baby that would never grow. I wept for myself. I wept for Steph and I was incredibly afraid that I would have to wait an absolute age before any doctor would let me go through treatment again. The doctors in England told me to stop taking the progesterone, a drug I was using as part of my fertility treatment to help stabilise a possible pregnancy and prevent miscarriage, but I'd been supplied with this by my doctors in

Belgium. They didn't really hold out any hope for my pregnancy either, but they thought that, in the grand scheme of things, continuing with the progesterone for an extra few weeks wouldn't really do me any harm. They thought we may as well wait until we were absolutely sure. I agreed and kept taking it, despite the contradictory advice.

I was told the danger signs to look out for with an ectopic pregnancy and I had to report any pain immediately. In the meantime, we would keep testing every three or four days. There was nothing else anyone could do. Until my HCG rose to above 1,000, there was no point in doing a scan. Even if a baby was there inside my womb, it would be too tiny to see.

I entered a period of emotional decline. I couldn't sleep, I couldn't work and I couldn't eat. My misery was intensified because I could not tell the people that I needed to understand what was wrong with me. Don't get me wrong. I was not left alone. I had counsellors galore and the nurses were great, even though, for my sake, they had to be realistic.

The potential media scrutiny was a huge problem. Journalists and well-wishers still enquired after my progress on a regular basis. They had been told absolutely nothing. They didn't even know I had had any treatment. Imagine the field day the newspapers would have had with this latest news: *Diane Blood's ectopic pregnancy and why she should never have been allowed to try for her husband's baby.* I could see the headlines now.

Not being able to share my problem with my closest friends made life very difficult during this crisis. My family knew, but sometimes it is necessary for those around you to understand what is happening, so that they too can give support and help. Like me, my mum tried to remain optimistic, but my dad thought we'd taken leave of our senses and that disobeying the English doctors' orders was the act of someone who was desperate and unrealistic. He later explained to me that this was because it brought back unwelcome memories of my mother's ectopic pregnancy, but at the time he appeared to think that I should cease treatment immediately. Stephen's family understood the implications less well and just waited to see what transpired. I spared them the finer details. It could only cause them pain and, unlike some of my friends, they could do nothing practical to help.

Once again, I looked like ending up with nothing. No baby, no friends and no job. I had rebuilt my business, but it was collapsing around my ears because I could not explain to colleagues in the industry why I needed their help. It is no use going for a nice long chat with a counsellor when, from a practical point of view, what you really need to be able to do is tell your client and/or some publisher that they don't stand a chance of getting your advertising copy next week. You'll probably be in hospital and they will need to give you an extended deadline so you can employ a freelancer (who you also cannot tell why you need their help). It was a total nightmare.

Medical advice suggested that, depending on the physical damage, I might not be able to return to work for up to six weeks. As for the mental upset, only I could gauge how long it would take to recover.

It just isn't possible to simply vanish out of circulation with no explanation to anyone. I started trying to frame some elaborate lie and thought that perhaps I could claim I had appendicitis. But I concluded that I just couldn't. I don't actually think I'm capable of carrying out such a hoax. Instead, I downloaded the entire contents of my work computer onto data tape and placed it an envelope with instructions to send it to a friend's advertising agency if I was suddenly taken ill. It had to be updated daily to include any new work and instructions. I was sinking fast. Already I could not meet the appointments and expectations people had.

I was supposed to be sitting my A level Law exam in under a month, but I couldn't think about revision. As for my friends, how do you explain that suddenly you don't want to book tickets to that theatre production you'd previously said looked great? How do you ask someone to take your turn at driving to the cinema for no apparent reason? You feel so distraught that you know you are a danger to yourself, your passengers and to other road users, yet you cannot say why you just don't feel up to it. How can you be made to live a lie without ever opening your mouth? This paradox is perfectly possible. I know; I have been there on more than one occasion. This time, I was sure that I couldn't live through it.

There was physical pain, but not the kind the nurses had described as a signal of an ectopic pregnancy. This was more like a bad case of homesickness, an aching, a longing that would not abate. I was in no danger of mistaking it for a burst fallopian tube, although I could not imagine any pain which could be worse than the one I was already experiencing. Even my GP, Dr Delaney, was frustrated at being unable to help. There were no pills he could prescribe for this one. Instead, he gave me a present from his wife. She lent me a gift her mother had given her – a miraculous medallion. It was a silver pendant depicting the Virgin Mary that had been blessed at Lourdes. I appreciated the thought. Others believed I didn't have a prayer of things working out OK. I just about still did.

The doctors had made provisional arrangements for my operation to remove the baby from my fallopian tubes at the Jessop Hospital for Women, but we hoped that, by my next blood test, my hormone levels might have risen enough to see something on a scan at my local fertility clinic. There was still one other remote possibility. I could have a foetal sac inside my womb, but no baby. The pattern of HCG levels meant this was unlikely, but obviously it would be better than confirming the pregnancy was outside my womb.

My HCG had remained below the magical 1,000 for two whole weeks following the initial pregnancy test. It seemed an eternity. The day of the scan arrived. The HCG had just topped the 1,000.

I was wearing the miraculous medallion on a chain wrapped around my wrist and I now held it tightly whilst I prayed, silently. *Please, God, I know that this is a hopeless wish, but please help my baby. Let it be all right. Don't let it have to die.*

Paula, the nurse who'd been so kind and considerate throughout, came to sit with me for a moment before I went in for the scan. I looked at her rather forlornly and asked, 'Is there any chance the baby might be all right and growing inside my womb after all?'

She smiled slightly and squeezed my hand, 'Well, I suppose there's always the one in a million.'

I was called in for the scan. I was accompanied by my mother, Paula and Ros, another nurse who'd looked after me. The doctor had a good look around. I could see the monitor, but I could detect nothing from the scan. What I did notice was Paula and Ros suddenly leaning forward. The doctor and nurses were smiling. Not only was the foetal sac safe inside my womb, it contained the beginnings of a tiny baby – a little white fleck in the centre of a small black oval. It didn't look much, but it meant the world.

With all the heartache I'd just been through, it was a further miracle that I'd come through it without having a miscarriage. Tears welled in my eyes, but I was told to be cautious. The foetus was much smaller than it should have been and they were still unsure the pregnancy would progress normally. I was booked in for another scan in a week's time.

I relaxed, but the warning meant there were no big celebrations. My mum and I stopped off at a small park on the way back from the clinic to phone my dad and Stephen's parents. Everyone remained cautious. My mum and I just sat there on the bench for ages, saying nothing, just smiling. I had a warm inner glow. I think that my mum did too. We did not need words to savour the moment.

One week later, there was a heartbeat. It was confirmed. My body contained a new life – my little one in a million. The glow radiated a little further, but still no euphoria. Despite beating even less favourable odds, this wasn't like winning the lottery. If I search to find a similar analogy, it was more like arriving at 32 and discovering you'd been born incredibly wealthy but had never realised it. The riches were still sitting there but could not be claimed for another seven and a half months – and that's if everything went well.

The odds of miscarriage in the first twelve weeks of pregnancy are one in five – roughly the same odds I'd overcome to get pregnant in the first place (disregarding the additional problems I'd faced with obtaining the sperm and the subsequent court case). Many people who conceive naturally lose their baby without ever having realised they were pregnant in the first place. The sad thing about assisted conception is that, even leaving aside the practical difficulties of establishing yet another pregnancy, because you know you are pregnant or potentially pregnant right from the moment of conception, early miscarriage hits so much harder. I was just over six weeks pregnant. The next six weeks were the longest six weeks of my life. Imagine Christmas Eve. You're five years old and far too excited to sleep. You also know that Santa won't bring you your presents whilst you're awake. If only you could make the hours move faster, it would soon be morning. Personally, I never saw Santa arrive so I must have been to sleep at some point, but that night seemed to last forever. If you multiplied those hours spent awake as a child on Christmas Eve and stretched them out to fill six weeks, you might begin to have some idea of how slowly the time crawled by for me. I wasn't pessimistic – just frightened. I wanted to get it over with.

I was exceptionally tired and my morning sickness also lasted throughout the day and night. I think that God has a sense of humour. I wanted to be pregnant, so he made sure I knew I was pregnant. In a way, it was all very reassuring, but I would rather have just known I was pregnant and felt well.

Not so reassuring were the period-type pains I experienced during those first few weeks. The books say these are perfectly normal, but I never knew whether the bad news was about to be delivered. Work and revising for my A level Law exam went totally to pot. I spent much of my time at my mother's, where she could deliver much-needed tender loving care, whilst I concentrated on knitting my first matinee jacket for the baby – about the most taxing activity I could contemplate.

The law exam came and went. It wasn't terribly important that I passed. I had decided to study for it to occupy myself and give myself the social contact afforded by an evening college course after my court case was over. I had been doing so much work for my case that I thought it unwise to suddenly stop and leave myself with nothing to do at night. Nevertheless, I did actually manage to pass, despite feeling compelled to leave a little early after one of the papers. I had this dreadful pain in my stomach and I needed to go and investigate the situation in the loo. No spots of blood. We were all right after all.

The media, at this point, were still an ever-present force in my life. They didn't have a clue that I'd had any treatment, but they were still waiting for some news and would call me regularly with various deals. I wasn't interested, but I knew they would have to be dealt with at some point. As my clinicians abroad were so keen to keep everything secret, I'd rather hoped to be able to go over at some point and hopefully they'd be able to think of a strategy that would work and we could agree on. Personally, I didn't have the energy to think about it.

I was ten weeks pregnant. Just two more weeks to go and then the worst would be over. I diverted myself with shopping for a new bathroom. I didn't have a shower in mine and decided that, with a new baby, a shower would be a necessity. I'd found the one I wanted in a showroom in Sheffield. I wanted to take my parents to see what they thought, so we went over one Saturday afternoon. It was an expensive purchase to be making, so there were lots of questions to ask. I wanted to get on and sort it out, but the showroom was busy and I stood waiting for ages. I really felt I needed to sit down. Again, I had an awful pain in my tummy, but I was learning not to worry so much.

My parents drove me back home and decided they would fetch a Chinese takeaway for tea. I didn't want one. I just wanted to sit down. They chose their meal, ordered it by phone from my house and then picked it up on their way home.

I felt awful. I sat huddled in a corner on my settee. The pain was bad. I fought the urge to get up, go to the loo and investigate, but in the end I had to. I just needed to check everything was all right.

It wasn't. There was blood everywhere. Even though I had suspected it, I still couldn't believe it. I thought perhaps if I quickly flushed away the evidence and went and sat back on the settee, perhaps it would all go away and we could pretend it hadn't happened. I didn't even reach for a sanitary towel. To do so would have been to admit it was all over. I was unconcerned about staining my clothes or the settee. What did it matter, if my baby had died?

I called my parents on my way back to the settee. They'd just finished their Chinese. They called the doctor and came immediately.

Now, I'm not stupid. I've read the books and I do know that spotting in early pregnancy is quite common and doesn't necessarily mean there's a problem. Most of these pregnancies continue normally, but this was a lot of blood. I hadn't noticed any clots, though, which was good. The doctor diagnosed a threatened miscarriage and thought my chances of remaining pregnant were around 50 per cent. Just when I thought the real worries were over, I was back to even odds. In days gone by, the doctor would have prescribed bed rest, but now the jury was out on whether it did any good. He left it up to me. Once the bleeding had stopped, I would need a scan to see if I was still pregnant.

I went to bed – and waited. This was my longest night. My mum stayed with me. I prayed for the bleeding to stop, but it continued all through the night and into the next morning. Gradually, throughout the day on Sunday the bleeding became less and by Monday morning it had finally stopped.

The start of the rest of my life

I went for my scan. Miraculously, the baby was still fine. Its little heart was pumping away. I was so relieved. I was supposed to have stopped taking my progesterone that weekend, but in view of what had just happened, I was told to continue with it until 12 weeks' gestation. There was almost a fortnight to go before we would finally see if my pregnancy could sustain itself without help.

The time elapsed without incident, so I started weaning off the progesterone as instructed. And then the next bombshell hit. Again, it was a Saturday afternoon. Only the week before, I'd turned down an offer from the *Sunday Times* of £10,000 for informing them of any pregnancy the day before anyone else. Now it was the *Sunday Times* again. They congratulated me on my pregnancy. I was flabbergasted, but I wasn't going to be shocked into revealing anything they didn't know for certain.

'I'm absolutely amazed . . . that you think I'm pregnant,' I faltered, trying to search for words that would imply denial without actually lying.

'We don't think, we know,' came the reply. Apparently, their health correspondent had learnt the news whilst attending a medical conference in Sweden the previous week.

Trying to think rapidly, I suggested that if it was the health correspondent that knew of this then perhaps she herself should give me a call. This was no time to be playing Chinese whispers. I was annoyed that the news had been passed on to someone else. I needed to know exactly how much the health correspondent knew and with what degree of certainty. She called me back straightaway and apologised for initially asking someone else to call.

It immediately became apparent that the game was up. They had the information which, the week before, had been worth £10,000 to them. She knew too much, including my approximate gestation. She wouldn't reveal her sources, other than that she had been told by three doctors at the conference. Two were from Belgium, one was from Denmark. I don't believe they meant any harm or realised the gravity of the news they had spilt. The doctors apparently now considered the risk of my pregnancy miscarrying to be over, which was nice to know. I was still worrying about my weekend weaning off the drugs. I don't think I actually told her anything at that point, other than that I needed time to think and that, if I was pregnant, I wouldn't deny it. I promised to call her back, but I didn't have long because her deadline was looming.

I called my parents for an emergency conference. I called Belgium, but only the cleaner answered the phone. She couldn't give me any emergency contact numbers for the weekend and told me I'd have to wait until Monday, which wasn't much use when we were talking about the Sunday newspapers. Naturally, she had no concept of the urgency of my situation.

We decided to put out an announcement on PA (the Press Association syndicate) confirming my pregnancy. I wished it hadn't become public so soon, but I could hardly deny it. The *Sunday Times* story was going front page, so they'd all know by the morning anyway and – as ever – the more exclusive the story, the bigger the splash. I didn't call the *Sunday Times* back, instead we just referred them to PA so everyone got the same story and no one could ask questions. They didn't have a problem with this.

So far, I had told only my own and Stephen's immediate family of my pregnancy. I had hoped to get time to tell my remaining family and friends before they heard the news from elsewhere. I was thwarted. The news was on TV before I had put down the telephone to PA and the press had already called my grandmother, who was probably thoroughly confused by the whole thing. She told them she didn't know what they were talking about.

The panic over, I faxed Belgium and bedded down for the night, knowing that I had no control over what would be printed in the morning papers. I would go out and buy them when I got up.

Some chance of that! The next morning, I was woken by someone hammering at the door. Not fancying the risk of getting photographed in my nightie, I hid under the duvet and hoped they'd go away.

They were persistent. I decided to get to a phone and call for help. The nearest phone was located in the spare bedroom at the front of the bungalow. I crawled into the room, so that I couldn't be seen through the curtains, and rang a neighbour. My neighbours had been great throughout and were very protective of me. I explained my predicament and they immediately went out and gave the offending journalist a piece of their mind. It worked, and soon all was quiet on the Western Front. Eventually, I mustered enough courage to peer through the curtains. Towards the bottom of the street a line-up of cars contained men with mobile phones lying in ambush. They weren't hassling me, but I was pretty well trapped.

The start of the rest of my life

I called my mum, who said she'd come and get me. I threw on some clothes, threw up (as per my normal morning routine) and then slipped out into the car with my mother.

When we reached the bottom of the street, the cars followed us. We called my father from the mobile, who told us not to lead the journalists to their house, so we tried to lose the cars en route to the park. This was something of a joke, as my mother rarely exceeds 20 miles an hour and certainly wasn't going to drive erratically with her pregnant daughter in the car. We took a wrong turn into a cul-de-sac and they followed us, turning around at the bottom of the street before doubling back to rejoin the main road. We almost lost them because there was quite a stream of traffic and they couldn't get out immediately behind us. Unfortunately, they soon caught us up again.

We finally lost them on a roundabout, doing about five miles an hour. Actually, I think they thought we were going to turn onto the A1. They headed back to Worksop, no doubt to cover my house. We continued to the park.

It was quite a pleasant morning to sit on a bench in a park, but after a while we began to realise that we couldn't stay there forever. Mobile phone calls to my neighbours, my father, my parents-in-law and Sue, my sister-in-law, quickly confirmed that journalists were waiting at our every possible port of call. We eventually chose the house with the smallest posse – Sue's.

A cup of tea and a few more phone calls later, we finally decided that really we had no choice, we would have to agree to do a short press conference, otherwise they weren't going to go away. We hastily arranged the venue – The Innings (the public house we'd used previously) – and we fixed the time for late afternoon. With everything arranged and the media placated, my mother and I finally felt safe enough to go back to my parents' home.

Photographers kept knocking at the door, trying to get their shots first in the exclusive setting of my parents' garden, but we told them to wait. One in particular had a huge sob story about wanting to get home to his wife and child. It was Sunday, after all, and he'd had no dinner. Neither had we. We told him to wait. I vaguely thought about trying to get home for a change of clothes and to put some make-up on, but I felt too ill to contemplate the car journey. I looked in the mirror. The lack of make-up wasn't as noticeable as it might have been. Pregnancy had given my skin a reasonably healthy glow, but I'd had a rough day chasing around. No wonder it was reported in the following day's papers that I looked tired.

The press conference was a civilised affair. Gill and Brian, Stephen's parents, had to cancel their planned evening out so that they could join us. They wanted everyone to know that they shared my joy. With all the reporters gathered together, no one wanted to be the one to ask anything intrusive. They were all delighted for me. They wanted to know when the baby would be born, what I planned to call my little one – the usual questions you might ask a friend on discovering that she was expecting. I was, after all, a normal expectant mother. My hopes and dreams were pretty much the same as anyone else's. I explained to them that I didn't want anything to cause me stress. The journalists seemed to understand and they promised that they would then leave me alone for the rest of my pregnancy.

After the press conference, the pub landlady invited us for a glass of champagne or (in my case) orange juice. The photographers were still around. They were processing their film and sending the images via modem to their various newsdesks. Even the photographer who was missing his food, wife and child was still around. He was happy to chat about the merits of digital technology and was no longer worried about getting home in a hurry.

The photographers wanted to photograph our mini celebration. I asked them not to. They didn't and everyone agreed that they hadn't seen us. I didn't want it to be reported because, to be honest, it didn't really feel very natural to me to be popping the champagne corks at that moment in time. It was nice chatting with the landlady, but, on the one hand, I knew I'd been pregnant for a while, and, on the other, I was still nervous that something would go wrong. As I commented previously, becoming pregnant was never a cause for momentary jubilation. It was more of a constant warm glow that left a smile on my face (when I wasn't being sick).

CHAPTER 18

Liam's birth

The books (which, by now, I'd read in great detail) claim that pregnancy sickness generally stops around the 12th to 14th week. My pregnancy was obviously never destined to conform to the normal rules. I passed these milestones with the sickness showing no signs of abating. In fairness, various potential remedies were on offer, but I wouldn't take them. I grew up in the days immediately following the Thalidomide disaster and a kid on our street had no ears. I'd put up with the sickness.

My first scan at the hospital was very heartwarming. My mum came with me. Obviously, I would have preferred to have been going with my husband, like most of the other expectant mothers, but I had known Steph wouldn't be there from before my child was conceived so that wasn't too upsetting. I was concentrating on the little one in my tummy. With all the problems I'd experienced, I'd obviously had plenty of scans before, but the scanners used at these early stages were not so detailed and the baby had not been so fully developed. This time I could make out the image of a tiny little baby. It was perfectly formed and wafting its arms around. I fell in love with it completely. This was my little fighter who had overcome such incredible odds to get this far. It was just as though it was waving at me, 'Hello, Mum. I know you're looking at me.'

I was offered various tests and asked to consider carefully whether I wanted them or not. I knew, however, that the answers could lead to even more difficult decisions and there is an argument that, at the end of the day, if you wouldn't take any action if potential problems are discovered, it might be better simply not to know. I'd had no hesitation about having the scan. They also offered to take a nuchal fold measurement to determine the risk of having a baby with Down syndrome and I agreed. The nuchal fold measurement was fine. The baby was also examined for signs of spina bifida. Everything looked normal.

I left the hospital clutching my little printout of the scan. I was very happy. I showed it to my dad and Steph's parents. The static image didn't have quite the same impact as seeing the baby move, but nonetheless everyone still expressed delight.

A couple of weeks later, the next test was on offer. The midwife takes a blood sample, again to determine the risk of Down syndrome and spina bifida. I felt I'd had enough of blood tests, with all the problems caused by knowing my HCG levels and being told my pregnancy was ectopic, so initially I declined this one, but I was later persuaded to change my mind. My GP seemed quite shocked that I'd declined the test. He told me that everyone normally has it and that he thought I ought to have it so I could be reassured that everything was all right. My father thought that this was very sound advice and so, in the end, I agreed to the test. The midwife came to my home to take the blood sample.

'Are you sure you really want this test?' she asked. She had been with me at the doctor's when we'd talked about the test and wanted to make sure that I was following my own wishes and not being pushed into doing something because of the views of others.

'Yes. Please take the blood sample,' I replied. Actually, I wasn't sure at all, but she was here in my home now so I could hardly change my mind again.

The sample was taken. I thanked the midwife and put it to the back of my mind. But, unfortunately, the test came back positive for Down syndrome. It identified a one in sixty chance that my baby would suffer from the problem. So much for the theory about being reassured that everything was fine. I was given another appointment at the hospital the following day to discuss my options.

I felt I had to tell my friends and family because it took the edge off my happiness and I needed them to understand. I was particularly gutted that lunchtime. Just after being told the test results, I went out for a pub lunch with my friend Helen. A couple of strangers bounced up to me and said, 'Oh, Mrs Blood.

Congratulations. We were so pleased to hear the news of your pregnancy. I bet you are just so excited.'

Normally, I would have been pleased that they were so happy for me, but this time I just wanted to blurt out my newly discovered problems. Of course I couldn't, so I thanked them and unburdened myself on my friend.

Helen was a great support. She listened without imposing her views, but the subject of potentially disabled unborn children is a highly charged subject and people have very strong opinions. As my child didn't have a father who could comment, everyone else seemed to feel it was their duty to tell me what they thought I should do. Actually, however, I was very sure of Stephen's opinion, if he had been alive. He didn't agree with abortion so he wouldn't have wanted me to investigate the situation further; but, as he wasn't here to help look after a child with special needs, he would have probably understood if I felt I needed to know more.

I did want to know if my child would be OK, and if there were going to be problems then I felt I'd rather know and have time to prepare for them. I am pretty sure I wouldn't have aborted an unhealthy child, although I don't think anyone can ever say for certain unless they are actually placed in the position of knowing their child will definitely be disabled.

Right now, I had three options. I could have an amniocentesis test, which carried a 1 per cent risk of miscarriage. I would know the result in two or three days. Taking a CVS (chorionic villus sample) carried possibly a very slightly higher risk of miscarriage, but I would know the next day. Alternatively, I could wait for the 20-week scan. At 20 weeks, they would also be able to examine the heart, which would probably be impaired in a child with a more severe case of Down syndrome, and they could also look for other clues. For instance, a child with Down syndrome has a knuckle on their little finger, but often they don't have a second joint nearer the end. They are also often smaller than average height, so their femur may be shorter.

At 20 weeks, there would still be time to do a CVS if further indicators were found, so I decided to wait. I was also reassured by a scan which was carried out there and then. The joint on the little finger could be seen and everything looked normal enough at that stage, although the heart wasn't really developed enough to examine.

If I'd had further tests and caused a miscarriage purely to put my mind at rest (or give me time to prepare for the worst), I would never have been able to forgive myself. It wasn't only the practical problems that I'd have trying to create another pregnancy, which your average couple would not face; I really wanted this child. No other would do. This was the one who'd overcome so much to wave their little arms at me at the last scan. How could I possibly put this fragile life at risk? I concluded that this baby needed me to protect them, whatever their problems may or may not be.

At the 20-week scan, all still looked well. The heart appeared to be normal, but the shadow of the positive Down syndrome blood test still hung over us. Again, I was offered the opportunity to have a CVS. I declined and got on with the business of trying to enjoy the rest of my pregnancy. This was not easy because I was still suffering from such awful pregnancy sickness and was having real problems with a heightened sense of smell. I'd already had to buy a new base for my bed because the old one suddenly smelt fusty, and my new leather bag had been consigned to the garage only days after purchasing it, as it made me retch every time I got near it. In the summer, it seemed to me that everyone had the most offensive body odour. Mind you, I couldn't stand the smell of soap either. Fortunately, grapefruit-scented soap came to the rescue. Grapefruit was OK. It was one of the few things I still liked to eat – in vast quantities.

Once the baby began to kick, I began to enjoy myself more. I liked the fluttering sensation and the reminder that my baby was alive, well and growing. On one visit to the doctor's, I commented to everyone that I thought my baby was going to be a footballer because my little one was so good at kicking. This caused quite a stir, as people suddenly presumed that I knew I was expecting a boy. Of course, I had no idea whether my baby was male or female. It was just a throwaway remark and, not for the first time, I found it quite amusing that such significance had been attached to my words.

Actually, if anything, I had been reasonably convinced that I was carrying a little girl. This was based on nothing more technical than a bunch of old wives' tales. My bump was all at the front. Most people seemed to think that this indicated a girl, although a few thought a bump at the front meant a boy and more evenly distributed weight indicated a girl. Everyone remembered the old wives' tale, but there seemed to be some confusion over which way round the story went. A wedding ring dangled on a hair over my stomach moved round in circles. This again supposedly indicated a girl. It was good fun to speculate, but I can't say I placed any faith in these two methods of determining the sex of a baby. A third method I felt more inclined to trust. It is statistically true that people who suffer from bad pregnancy sickness are more likely to have a girl. It's something to do with the hormones. On this basis, my baby should definitely have had two X chromosomes.

I wasn't really bothered which sex my baby was, though, at times, I thought I might have a slight preference for a girl. This view remained from when we were trying for the baby before my husband died. I still planned to call her Shannon, the name that Steph and I had chosen together, followed by Stephanie, the feminine form of my late husband's name. But I felt that I would also like a boy, especially now my husband was no longer around. I thought it would be nice to have someone to carry on the family name.

Whenever I dreamed about the baby, it was always a boy. In a vivid dream I had had the night the baby was first conceived, Steph visited me in my hotel bedroom. I kept asking him questions, but he appeared unable to talk. Instead, he took a piece of paper and drew on it. He began, 'I ♡ . . .' I had expected him to continue with U, but instead he drew a person. I thought he must be drawing me, but it turned out to be a boy. More recently, I'd dreamt about the birth. What was once a distant dream was now something I could really begin to plan for and look forward to.

The highlight of my pregnancy was a trip to London for the Baby and Child Show at Earls Court in early October. This couldn't have been a bigger contrast to the year I had visited the same exhibition just a few days after my first court hearing. We made a real treat of the occasion, with myself, my mother and my cousin Julie staying over for a few days in a hotel. The show provided a great opportunity to decide on all my baby essentials. I was still being recognised almost everywhere I went and everyone was so pleased for me. One company, Bébécar, offered to give me the pram I had selected. I also chose a cot and, in between it all, I managed to do a little work. In the evening, we took in one of the London shows, *Whistle Down the Wind*. I couldn't remember the last time I'd been so happy. Finally feeling confident enough to choose things for my baby really brought it all home to me. That dream of our child, which my husband and I had discussed so long ago, was nearly a reality. I wished that he could have shared the excitement of those days, but I was sorry for Steph, not for myself. I had taken on our child with no expectation of a husband's support, so I didn't feel cheated in the same way as I imagine I might have if we had conceived in the natural way and then he had tragically died at some point between the conception and the birth.

Although I would probably do less work once the baby arrived, I had always planned to continue working for my company once we had a family. In that sense, being a single-parent family would make no difference. OK, we would only have one income, but Steph had worked so hard to provide for our family before he died and we'd had a standard endowment policy for the value of our mortgage. I was lucky that I could do most of my work from home. In fact, I was just lucky full stop. I couldn't imagine it being possible to be any happier.

The next few weeks were very precious. I was still being sick on a daily basis, but the nausea wasn't quite as bad as it had been. I could feel my baby kicking and reacting to almost every move. We particularly enjoyed bathtime, when the baby liked to do somersaults in my tummy. The baby calmed when it heard music, especially when I sang. I held little one-way conversations with my bump and I really began to feel we were getting to know each other. I also started my six weeks of parentcraft lessons. My cousin Julie attended the first one with me, as she planned to be with me for the labour. We thought that everyone else would be accompanied by their husbands, but in the majority of cases the husband was at work, so most women went alone. At the lessons, we talked about pain relief for the labour and I decided that I would like to use a TENS machine, which uses tiny little electrical currents to help release the body's natural pain-relieving hormones. I could borrow one from the Jessop Hospital, where I was booked in for the birth, so I made an appointment there to learn how to use it.

I never made it to the appointment and only completed my first few weeks of parentcraft lessons, however, as things started to go wrong. I had a couple of days when I was in terrible pain. It would come on slowly, build to a crescendo of almost unbearable proportions and then fade quickly. It didn't feel like contractions, more like bad period pain, all down my right-hand side and into my back. The midwife came to check it out and we consulted the doctor, but everyone was baffled. I began to be really worried that I must have a low pain threshold. If I was suffering like this with the preliminaries, I wondered how on earth I would get through labour.

I went to stay at my parents' house, so they could look after me. I spent most of my time in the bath, as it was the only way I could get any relief from the pain. The doctor diagnosed a kidney infection and prescribed antibiotics. I hadn't taken any drugs at all, all the way through my pregnancy, apart from the progesterone, but right now I would have taken anything. I just had to stop the pain.

I eagerly waited for the antibiotics to do their stuff, but several days later they'd had no effect whatsoever. Finally, one night I could stand it no longer. I'd had about as many baths as my wrinkled skin could take and I really thought that the situation needed to be investigated in hospital. It was the middle of the night and so we travelled the short distance to Bassetlaw, our local hospital, instead of going all the way to the Jessop Hospital, where I was to give birth, in Sheffield. In any event, we'd agreed with the midwives at the Jessop that I would check that I was in labour before turning up on their doorstep. This was in order to avoid any unnecessary risk of publicity surrounding the birth.

At Bassetlaw Hospital, I saw a doctor who confirmed that I wasn't experiencing labour pains; they gave me some painkillers and booked me in for the night, but the pain didn't let up. By now, it was a constant undulating ache, so I was kept in for observation. I did discover that if I lay permanently on my left-hand side, I could relieve it somewhat. This was fine until, say, for example, I wanted to eat, drink or be sick (which, unfortunately, still usually featured somewhere in my daily schedule). I couldn't even bear to sit up for a few minutes.

I was at least reassured that they could try and monitor the baby's heart on a daily basis, but I could only stand the machine to be applied for a few seconds. I desperately wanted to lie still, but the pain forced me to move and then I felt guilty because it was my fault they couldn't get a proper CTG (cardiotocograph) foetal monitoring trace. This went on for a few days, with aborted attempts at tracing the baby's heart a couple of times a day. I didn't really think that the baby was in distress or suffering problems associated with its heart, so initially I wasn't too worried – as long as we had at least confirmed it ticking away for a few seconds. After all, that's all I would get at this stage if I wasn't in hospital and I was here because of my pain, which was supposed to be a kidney infection and nothing to do with the baby at all. We had also done a quick scan with a portable machine. The baby and placenta, which was attached to the right-hand wall of my womb, looked fine.

To be honest, I thought that if I could lie completely still, drink from a straw and not move from my left-hand side for the next four and a half weeks until the baby was due, all would be well. My father, however, worried about my lack of movement. With my mother having suffered a pulmonary embolism, he feared that my blood might clot if I remained so inactive. The concerns began to grow.

One night, a new midwife was on duty. She introduced herself as Joanne and did the usual unsuccessful routine of trying to get a trace on my baby's heart. After a short while, she returned saying that she had read my notes and the consultants really needed us to persevere and get a longer trace. By endurance, patience and a willingness on her part to hold the monitors by hand, we eventually got what they were looking for.

It was really late at night and I snuggled down in my bed, pleased we'd finally got what they needed to check my baby was well. I was just nodding off, when the midwife returned with a doctor. She had shown him the trace and they were worried the baby's heartbeat was so low. They wanted another trace. More pain and frustration later, as I still couldn't hold still, they managed to get a further short trace and the doctor said he was satisfied until the morning when they'd order a Doppler scan to measure the blood supply going to the baby. So much for my night's sleep. I lay awake worrying all night.

The next morning, we tried for the scan. They saw the baby and it was moving around, but we couldn't measure the blood supply, again because I just couldn't lie still and also because the baby was so active.

They gave up, saying, 'A baby that active can't be having any problems.'

I was still concerned and I felt so guilty. I wished I could have kept still. My father asked for a doctor to come and see me and explain the results of my scan. Basically, he just told me that the scan operator was satisfied, even though they couldn't measure the blood supply and, in any case, it was all largely irrelevant because it was too early to deliver the baby by Caesarean.

I began to feel that being in hospital was a complete waste of time. Even if something was wrong, it seemed they couldn't do anything about it. I thought I may as well go home, which they agreed to, as long as I had stopped worrying. I hadn't, of course, but I wouldn't worry any more for being at my parents' home. Also, I would no longer be able to hear the screaming of other women giving birth. My room at Bassetlaw was positioned around a courtyard. The labour ward was at right angles to my room and sometimes it got really loud. I began to wonder how I would fare when it was my turn.

It was the morning of Friday, 11 December. I had been booked to go to a Publicity Association Christmas party with work that afternoon. I'd decided I'd better call that off, but we began making plans for me to go home, arranging for my parents to come and collect me by car. I was waiting for them to arrive when someone came to tell me that an appointment had been made for me to see my consultant at the Jessop Hospital early that afternoon. Apparently, my GP was still worried, even if I wasn't, and he'd called and asked them to see me. My parents were still coming to collect me, but we'd only have time for a quick sandwich before shooting over to Sheffield.

We called at my parents' home briefly. I made a quick phone call for work, but we were running late so we had to skip the sandwich. The journey to Sheffield had a rather strange sense of déjà vu about it. The last time I could remember noticing so many bumps in the road was the time we had taken Steph to Sheffield in the ambulance. It felt rather ominous.

I complained to my dad, 'Please can you try and not hit so many bumps.'

'Well, it's up to you. We can either get there quickly or you can have a smooth ride. Which would you prefer?'

It was the same answer as three and a half years earlier. 'Both.'

My dad dropped my mother and me off at the hospital door, before going to look for somewhere to park. He joined us as soon as he could. We had just about made it to the appointment on time.

I explained the problems I'd been having to the consultant and the midwife tried to do another trace on the baby's heart. As usual, it took two or three attempts to get anything like a reasonable length of trace. Fortunately, she was very patient. I kept having to break off and go and lie on my left-hand side until the pain subsided and I could bear to try again. Eventually, the machine blipped to say that my baby had reached the requirements for the machine to consider it was OK. The midwife disagreed with the machine. She said that, whilst it was not overly concerning, it wasn't exactly a normal, healthy trace either.

We progressed on to another attempt for a Doppler scan. The consultant was busy explaining things to me, but by that time I was completely out of it. I was in so much pain trying to lie on my back that I haven't a clue whether they saw anything helpful or not.

It was decided that the best thing was to admit me to the ward, whilst they tried to get another trace on the baby's heart. In the meantime, I was to sift my urine, looking for these supposed kidney stones that were causing me so much grief. I spent a lot of time in the toilet. The pain was so bad that I felt I had to do something and I hoped that emptying my bladder might relieve it. Of course, that theory only holds true if your bladder is full in the first place. Mine never got the chance.

Being admitted to the Jessop in such a hurry had sent security arrangements into disarray. We were worried about my own and the baby's safety, both from the media and from potential nutters. I had received one particularly threatening letter with the announcement of my pregnancy, so we took the view that we couldn't be too careful. Most maternity wards nowadays have locks and cameras on every door, but the Jessop Hospital was built in an age when such precautions weren't necessary. They had baby tags and I dare say they would have installed other security were it not for the fact that the hospital was scheduled to be closed down in a couple of years. The new one was already being built.

They decided to open up a ward that had been closed down for Christmas. It was opposite the general maternity ward, sharing the same landing and nursing office. It meant that I would be all on my own, but the ward had a separate digital lock on the door and it was re-programmed with a number that my family specified. We could all get in and out, but there was no risk of anyone else already knowing the number. It also meant that my family could come and go at any time without us disturbing the rest of the patients and generally disrupting the usual running of the hospital. I had my own day room, my own shower and toilet block at the end of the ward, and my own payphone. All of this may sound like very special treatment, and it was, but these were very special circumstances. It wasn't just the security. My parents might not be able to visit at conventional hours. They would be too busy running the gauntlet of the media posse. We would also have to be able to discuss how to deal with them – in private. Fortunately, nearly all the beds at the Jessop Hospital maternity ward were in their own little room, so it had always been planned that I could have a private room. The private ward was a bit of a Christmas bonus.

I was now under the care of a different midwife – the one on the maternity ward. She was trying to get an adequate trace on my baby's heart in between looking after all the other patients in maternity. It was hopeless. Every time she tried, I ended up in agony. I was also starving. I still hadn't had any lunch and it was late afternoon. Eventually, my parents managed to get me a chocolate bar to eat and, after more discussions with the consultant, the midwife decided to give me some pethidine. It wasn't ideal. It could make the baby sleepy, which might in itself lead to an abnormally slow heart trace. It was, however, the only viable option. They needed to control my pain enough for me to remain still.

When considering my birth plan (I'd never actually got round to writing it), pethidine hadn't exactly been a favoured option of mine. Come to think of it, not much was, although I'd begun to revise my thinking after I'd heard the screaming sessions at Bassetlaw Hospital. Before that, I was one of these first-time mums who was going to be an absolute martyr, surviving on gas and air, a TENS machine and determined to enjoy every minute of the experience. I thought that pethidine would probably make me feel nauseous and not have much effect on the pain, but I take back everything. It worked really quickly and it was absolutely wonderful to be free of pain. I sat quite still whilst the midwife traced the baby's heart for almost an hour. I looked at her for a reaction to what she was seeing, but she didn't give a lot away. She predicted that it was a boy, because boys usually have a slower heart rate and she told me that she thought the baby was asleep. No surprise there, then.

She kept disappearing and then coming back for another look. I suspected that she was discussing the results with the consultant, but it wasn't until she asked if I'd had anything to eat that day that I began to suspect what they were thinking. She would rather I hadn't just eaten the chocolate bar, but they'd work round it.

The consultant came in to see me. He was supposed to be going on holiday that night, but he'd stayed late to see me. He explained my options. It wasn't clear that the baby was definitely in distress, but the trace was abnormal and the heart rate had been consistently low for a long time, even if we disregarded the results I'd reported from Bassetlaw. He recommended an emergency Caesarean, although I could wait until something clearer happened, which would force them to act. He thought that if my baby was born now, at 36 weeks to the day, it would fare quite well. The only difficulty might be its breathing, as the lungs wouldn't be fully developed.

I wanted to know about the heart.

'No, that would be OK.'

When was the consultant back off holiday?

'In a week's time.' His colleagues would take good care of me in the meantime.

I thought about it for a second and then decided that the baby needed to be born. It seemed my body had been telling me that all was not well for long enough.

The consultant looked very relieved. I was surprised that he already had the consent form for the operation in his hand. 'You just need to sign here,' he pointed.

He had obviously thought that I didn't really have much choice after all. 'I think you're doing the right thing. I don't think I could have slept tonight knowing that baby was still inside your womb.'

All my carefully laid plans for the birth had suddenly gone awry. 'I haven't got my camera,' I complained to my parents. I didn't have any clothes or nightwear either, but I didn't really care about that. I wouldn't get another chance for the photo.

My parents promised to get the camera and started discussing who to call. I, meanwhile, was already being wheeled to theatre. The staff came running from all directions. I was surprised they were running. I perhaps had still underestimated the urgency of my situation. I'd hit them bang on clocking-off time, but they told me that they were delighted to stay and be of assistance at the birth of such a precious baby.

People began explaining various things that were to happen. I was in such a whirl that the whole lot just floated over my head. I tried not to worry and concentrated on 'enjoying' my birth experience. If this was how it was going to be, I didn't want my memories and feelings marred or wiped out by panic. We would have been in theatre sooner, but just as I was about to go in another lady whose need was more urgent than mine got pushed to the front of the queue. I wouldn't have noticed, if they hadn't told me. It was over so quickly anyway and I don't know who operated on her. It seemed to me that I had the full complement of staff fussing after me. The anaesthetist made small talk, asking me if I'd decided on names. I told him that I still hadn't made my mind up if it was a boy.

'Oh, well, that's it then. It's bound to be a boy,' he joked.

Soon we got the green light and all systems were go. My mother, my cousin Julie and my camera all came into the theatre for the birth. My GP wanted to be there, too, so he waited outside with my father. I was told that Gill, my mother-in-law, was on her way. Unfortunately, her husband Brian was en route to the airport, taking Stephen's youngest sister, Bev, and her husband back to their home in Germany. They couldn't be contacted.

My GP and the consultant exchanged a quick few words as I was wheeled into theatre. It seemed they had both been very worried about me. The consultant confirmed, 'I think it was a very sick lady in Bassetlaw Hospital this morning.'

My GP smiled, pleased that he'd done the right thing in ringing to get me an appointment at the Jessop. 'Well, we'll soon know whether it's a girl or a boy.'

'I already know,' the consultant retorted.

I was manhandled into position. The epidural meant that from the waist down I couldn't do a lot to help myself, although I wasn't entirely numb. The whole thing seemed to have had a bit of a lopsided effect as, due to my pain, they'd had to inject my spine whilst I was lying on my left-hand side. It felt as though all the anaesthetic had gravitated to that side and it had less sensation than the other. I voiced my concerns, but they proved to me that it had worked fine before erecting a green screen and beginning the job in hand. There was a lot of tugging and pulling. It was a bit uncomfortable, but I was determined to 'enjoy' it. Julie told me afterwards that I had a stupid fixed grin on my face. It wasn't entirely false. I was happy that I would soon have my baby with me and I was looking forward to learning its sex. A bit more tugging and pulling, and I began to panic. I complained to the anaesthetist that I could still feel far more on my right-hand side. Like a shot, he injected something into my right wrist and I was sent somewhere on cloud nine for an instant holiday.

The same man was also giving me a running report on what they could see as they pulled the baby from my womb.

'Loads of dark hair,' was the first thing I learnt about my little bundle. 'And can you remember what we were saying about the name?'

I couldn't. At this stage of the proceedings, anything more complicated than monosyllables was completely beyond me. I looked blank.

'It's a boy. You've got a little boy.'

It was 8.13 p.m. I heard him cry as they lifted him from my tummy. I was very relieved. I thought he must be OK if he could cry.

They quickly wrapped him up and held him in my arms very briefly. I couldn't really hold him entirely myself because the stuff they'd zapped into my wrist still left me a bit numb. I know it's a bit clichéd and that every mother thinks that theirs is the most beautiful baby in the world, but I really thought he was so handsome. His lips were a vibrant red and slightly pouting. He had a mass of dark hair and he looked at me briefly with big blue eyes veiled by long dark lashes. In hindsight, he looked a lot like my husband, but I never really got to grips with comparing babies' appearances to adults and, with everything that had just happened, I was too busy concentrating on my baby to afford the luxury of thinking too much about Stephen at that particular moment.

I thought my baby looked a bit Celtic. When Steph and I had gone on our last holiday together to my cousin's wedding in Ireland, the groom had been called Liam. Steph had never heard the name before and commented that he liked it, so that's the name I chose – Liam – Liam Stephen.

Liam Stephen had stopped crying and was making a funny snoring-type noise. I was a bit alarmed, but the midwife seemed calm. She explained that the noise was because my baby was having difficulty breathing and they were going to take him to the Special Care unit.

My dad and Gill caught only a brief glimpse of Liam as he passed on his way to Special Care. Gill cried with happiness when she was assured that the baby just needed a little help for now and would be OK. Nothing could replace her son, but here was the child he had wished for – her third grandson.

I was sad that Liam and I had to be parted so soon. I was wheeled out of theatre into the recovery room and they told me that my baby weighed 5 lb 13 oz, which I thought was quite respectable when he was four weeks premature. They promised to bring me a Polaroid picture of him soon and told me that I could go and see him in the morning.

Before I got my picture, the press were already on the phone.

'*The Sun* newspaper is calling reception. They've heard about the birth. What should we tell them?'

CHAPTER 19

Special Care for a very special baby

I left handling the press completely up to my dad. I couldn't be bothered to think about them. My parents and Stephen's mum all went to see Liam in Special Care. He was lying naked on his tummy in an incubator filled with oxygen. I was really concerned about his health, but everyone assured me that he was just in there for observation. He'd probably be back with me on the ward in the morning.

Our visitors left for the evening. I tried to sleep, but it was awful. I hated being parted from Liam and I was so worried. The snoring-type noise he had been making reminded me of the noise Stephen made just before his breathing arrested and he'd suffered the heart attack. I wished Liam was back in my tummy. At least that way we were together and I would know he was all right when he kicked. Now I had to rely on other people to reassure me that he was still hanging on in there. Every time a nurse came in to see me, I asked her to ring Special Care for a progress report. Unfortunately, there wasn't a lot anyone could tell me. Liam's condition hadn't changed and the registrar had gone to bed.

At just gone midnight I did receive one bit of good news, but it didn't concern Liam. Alison, the wife of my barrister, Michael Fordham, had also been expecting a baby. Our expected delivery dates were six weeks apart, but their baby had been overdue. There was still no sign of Alison going into labour when my father had rung to give Michael the news about Liam at around 10 p.m., but some time between then and midnight, Alison had given birth to a little girl: Lois. It was amazing that our children would share the same birthday.

The next morning was not good. Everyone told me that I felt so bad because I had baby blues. I thought this was a complete load of rubbish. I was, quite simply, worried sick. If Liam had been well, I would have been fine.

A nurse from Special Care came to see me first thing to explain his condition. He was very poorly. They were going to put him on CPAP (continuous positive airways pressure). They explained that this was not quite as severe as full ventilation, but that a continuous stream of air-oxygen mixture would be pushed through a pipe fed in through his nose so that his lungs wouldn't deflate.

'He will be all right, though, won't he? He's going to live?' I asked.

She didn't answer immediately. 'I would say his chances are 95 per cent. Yes.'

I was gutted. What about the other 5 per cent. What had I done? Why had I dragged him out into the world too soon? He might have been well and quite content where he was in my womb. It hadn't been obvious when they'd opened me up what had caused the problem with the low heart rate, but there were two possibilities. The umbilical cord had been trapped between Liam's head and my cervix. This didn't necessarily explain either my pain or the abnormal trace, but it did mean that we were lucky I hadn't gone into labour naturally. Unless the cord had moved, Liam would have pushed it out into the world in front of him and it would have torn from the placenta. This should have given me comfort that I had done the best thing, but it didn't. I just rationalised that I could have still left him another couple of weeks. Hindsight is a wonderful thing. It's a pity we can't tap into it whenever we want.

The other possibility could have been more immediately lethal. There had been a small blood clot behind my placenta. Was this a new wound or had it been there for some time? We didn't know. There were no real answers.

The only thing I can be sure of is that my pain had been caused by the pregnancy and not by my kidney. The consultant performing the Caesarean had a quick, non-expert look at my kidney whilst he was in there and said that it looked fine, which seemed to make sense. I was pumped full of painkillers because of the operation and the effects of the epidural were only just beginning to wear off, but I could no longer feel the pain I had experienced before. It had been so intense that, had the problem remained, I was sure I would still feel something, despite all the drugs. Thankfully, the pain never returned.

I was eager to see Liam, so the nurse got me into a wheelchair and wheeled me up to see him before they put him on CPAP, when my view would be obscured because of all the tubes and the little knitted hat he would have to wear. He was situated just next to the door on Intensive Care. He looked so helpless. He was panting fifty to the dozen and he looked exhausted.

I sat at the side of the incubator, stroking the glass, with tears rolling down my cheeks. 'I just want to breathe for him and give him a rest.'

'I know, but you can't. He's got to get better himself,' the nurse sympathised.

'When will that be? When will he be better?' I cried.

'We don't know. Maybe a couple of days.'

My visiting time was over. They told me that I needed to rest and recover from my own operation. I felt fine. It was just my little baby I was worried about.

My parents didn't get to visit until late morning. I kept ringing to try and get them over, as I desperately wanted to be comforted. They couldn't come just yet. The press had kept them up until 4 a.m. and a man from the *Daily Mail* was sitting in their lounge, so we couldn't have a proper conversation to explain what was wrong. I was very frustrated, because it seemed to me that my parents thought the biggest problem was the media. The man from the *Daily Mail* apparently thought that the biggest problem was that I couldn't put Steph's name on Liam's birth certificate. They wanted to know what I intended doing about it. But I knew the biggest problem was Liam's health. At that moment in time, I couldn't give a stuff about anything else, but then again I hadn't been kept up with the phones ringing until 4 a.m.

I am sure that my parents must have felt frustrated as well at not being able to talk or visit sooner, but they did not appreciate just how ill my little baby was. We all hear of babies who have been born prematurely. Usually by the time we know about it they have recovered with no ill effects. It is rare that you hear about the ones who weren't so lucky. Comparatively speaking, 36 weeks wasn't that early. No one expected my baby to be as poorly as he was. The previous night we had been led to believe that the breathing problems were very short-term. On that basis, my dad had assured me that Liam would probably be with me in the morning. My parents had no reason to suspect that things had changed.

They eventually arrived, having run the gauntlet of the press waiting outside the hospital. They decided to do a press conference at the hospital with Professor Cooke to try and answer some of the media's questions. I declined to participate. I was still in too much of a state and, besides which, the effect of the epidural hadn't worn off.

Some members of the media seem to leave their brains behind them when they're in pursuit of a story. GMTV had wanted both Liam and me in London, talking to them on a settee that morning. I'd just had major surgery and my son was in Special Care. It seemed to me that this small detail had washed over everyone's heads and it upset me. It felt as though the whole world was having a party because of us. We were too ill to go and they wouldn't wait until we were better. I already had floods of congratulatory cards and letters pouring in from the public. I was grateful, but I couldn't read them whilst Liam was ill. I'd look when he was better.

In the meantime, all four of Liam's grandparents opened the letters and cards for me. There were so many I'd never have got through them all myself anyway. We started displaying some of the cards, but there were too many so we just had to pile them up. In the end, they totalled almost 600. Even with the whole ward to myself, I was running out of space. In any case, every available surface was already covered with flowers.

Liam was totally oblivious to the fuss he had caused. Bless him. He was only concerned with trying to get his next breath and there was nothing much I could do to help. Puts everything into perspective, doesn't it? My sole job as a mother at that time was to try and express milk. Liam's stomach couldn't take milk just yet, but we hoped to freeze it for when he was ready. I had always wanted to breastfeed and, also, premature babies have more difficulty digesting formula milk, so it's important to build up a supply of their mother's milk, but I was failing miserably. I'd tried all the machines. I'd spoken to the breastfeeding advisers. I'd tried hand expressing and my poor small breasts had been pummelled and pulled in every way possible. At the end of a 45-minute session, I'd be rewarded with a tiny little drop of creamy-looking stuff in the bottom of a small jar. I'd label it up, with details of the time, date and who it was for, and then put it in the fridge. The nurses encouraged me that at least I was getting something, but it was very disheartening. It took such a long time and I was having difficulty fitting in expressing milk between my visitors and visiting Liam myself. For every tiny drop of breast milk I lovingly took to the ward fridge, Supermum (obviously somewhere else on the other maternity ward) had at least three full jars labelled up for her child. I spoke to the nurses about my concerns. They told me that I shouldn't compare. I was very anxious and I had had a difficult time. This could affect my milk supply.

Whenever I went to see Liam, I had no such problem. My milk would flow out all over my nightdress. It seemed such a shame I couldn't catch it, but I never seemed to have a container with me at the time and I would have been in full view of all the other visitors to Special Care.

The nurses on Special Care suggested I look at Liam's photo when expressing, but the Polaroids I had of him were not very good and looking at them didn't increase my milk supply. Then the nurses gave me a blanket which Liam had been lying on. The smell helped. I knew that the strong sense of smell I'd developed during pregnancy must be for a reason. Even through the bleach, I could definitely smell Liam. It was such a sweet smell, quite distinctive from any other baby. It was a shame I couldn't leave the port holes to Liam's incubator open longer. If I disinfected my hands first, I was allowed to open them to stroke the soft downy hairs on Liam's shoulders and to take in his wonderful fragrance, but I was told that it was better not to. I therefore rationed myself quite harshly, even though not being able to touch him was almost unbearable. It reminded me of the stong desire to touch my husband's skin when I had been prevented from doing so due to his illness.

It was Sunday before I was allowed to change Liam's nappy for the first time. I couldn't remember ever changing a baby's nappy before. I never expected my first attempt to be hampered by wires, an incubator and severe nerves. I would have been OK if it had been someone else's child, but Liam was so fragile and every time I moved, the alarms went off on his monitors. In the end, the nurse had to disconnect his heart monitor whilst I finished the nappy.

Special Care for a very special baby

That made me even more nervous. What if his heart stopped just at that moment and no one knew? It had already stopped once. I'd screamed at the nurses to come and help him. They wandered over quite serenely, calmly patted Liam on the bottom and off his heart went again as if there'd never been a problem.

'Aren't you concerned?' I asked.

'No,' they replied. 'They just do that sometimes. You get used to it.'

I hoped I wouldn't have to get used to it with Liam. It had nearly given me a heart attack, let alone Liam. When my husband's heart had stopped for a second, it had taken an electric shock to start it again.

I was beginning to get very concerned that Liam's health didn't seem to be improving. In fact, if anything, he'd got worse. His oxygen requirements had increased considerably, yet from what they had first said when Liam was born, I had expected him to be better by now. I wasn't quite sure whether everyone had just thought it kinder at the time to tell me that he'd be well in a few days or whether they really had expected him to recover sooner. I was very worried that he was not progressing as the doctors expected. The nurses assured me that he would get better and that they wouldn't lose him, but I'd heard that one before. When they did the brain scan on Stephen, they told me that he would get better, too.

The similarities between Stephen's final few days and Liam's first few were quite distressing. All were spent in Intensive Care. The crisis that had led to admission in each case was breathing difficulties. Also, both Liam and Steph had had brain scans (which were fine) and wires and tubes were attached to just about every organ. I was becoming far too expert at reading all the monitors. I was so afraid that Liam wouldn't make it. Professor Cooke explained to me that it was perfectly normal to feel like that. It was the body's way of preparing just in case the worst should happen. It didn't mean that it was at all likely. Even so, it was difficult to rationalise that I was being over-anxious, because I had been there before and Steph had died.

My biggest fear was that they would have to fully ventilate Liam. They had ventilated Stephen and never managed to get him to breathe again unaided. I wanted Liam to keep fighting on his own. I didn't want the same thing to happen to him. I didn't want him to become reliant on a machine and then not be able to function without it. I explained this to the paediatricians who were taking care of Liam. They assured me that they would never ventilate unless it was absolutely necessary, as this type of ventilation can sometimes cause long-term problems. It is so severe that the force of the oxygen being pushed into the lungs can sometimes pop the delicate little buds in the lung. It is a question of balance. Sometimes a baby just needs a rest and if you continued to let them struggle on alone, they would either burst their lung or just give up altogether.

Twice during Liam's time in Intensive Care the paediatricians told me that Liam had reached the point where they would have to fully ventilate. They assured me that it would just be for a short while. I was not so sure and I regurgitated my fears because of my experience with Stephen. On both occasions I left Liam, expecting him to be on full ventilation by the time I returned. I went up to my room and prayed that somehow Liam would pull through the crisis and that they wouldn't have to ventilate him after all. I'm not sure whether it was my prayers or the paediatricians' appreciation of the distress that full ventilation would cause me, but they held out before taking the action they had already told me was inevitable. Both times, Liam's breathing suddenly improved. He was never fully ventilated.

My lowest point was reached on the Monday morning after he was born. I woke with an urgent need to see Liam, but I was told that I couldn't visit because there was some kind of crisis in Special Care. I was scared to death that it was Liam who had suddenly taken a turn for the worse. I pestered the nurses on the ward to ring and enquire about him, but no real information was forthcoming. I was just told that Special Care would call when I could go up. I hovered around for ages waiting for the phone call, but in the end I was beside myself with worry. I phoned my parents, but they weren't in. They were calling at my home before making their way over to the hospital. I had no one to talk to and I wanted to be as near to my baby as possible. Despite my instructions to the contrary, I went up to Special Care and asked to wait in their waiting room. As it turned out, I think it was the best thing I could have done. If I'd stayed by myself any longer, I'm sure I would have driven myself insane.

A couple of mothers were already waiting to see their children in the Special Care waiting room. They were visiting from outside the hospital, so, unlike myself, they had nowhere else to sit. It was like a breath of fresh air chatting to them, even if it was potentially rather dangerous. They recognised me instantly and told me about all the journalists waiting outside the hospital. I was aware that they could tell them on the way out that they had been speaking to me and relay what they had learnt both about myself and my son, but I decided that at some point you just have to allow yourself to share your fears like any 'normal' mother and cease to worry about potential leaks of confidence. We chatted enthusiastically about our respective children and the problems they'd faced since birth. It was great to know that I wasn't the only person to have felt the way I did and also encouraging to know that one of their babies was improving.

Perhaps Liam would be better soon. I also learnt that the paediatricians were doing their rounds and it was not unusual to be locked out of Special Care for a period of time on a Monday morning. These women had been visiting Special Care for longer than me and were more used to the routine. It was just unfortunate that this particular morning the crisis I'd been told about (which turned out to have been a very sick baby being admitted) had been followed immediatcly by the normal rounds, which no one had mentioned.

Talking not only calmed my fears, it also helped to pass the time and soon we were allowed onto the ward. The nurse announced my arrival to those in Special Care, 'Liam's mum is here to see him.'

It was great being referred to as Liam's mum. I'd been Diane Blood for so long: Diane Blood's going to court, Diane Blood's won her appeal, Diane Blood's pregnant, the media want to talk to Diane Blood. A friend of mine had a four-year-old son who couldn't get to grips with the fact that I had a Christian name and a surname like everyone else. Every time I'd been on TV, his grandmother had told him to come and look, 'Diane Blood's on the TV.' As far as he was concerned, that was my sole title – both names rolled into one.

Liam was still very poorly and hadn't improved at all since my last visit. I told the nursing staff how concerned I'd been and asked if I could see one of the paediatricians in private. I decided that I needed some answers because I couldn't carry on the way I'd been that morning. The paediatrician fixed a time to come and see me in my room on maternity and duly arrived later that morning.

It was really helpful speaking to him. Liam had been more poorly than anyone had expected for a baby of his gestation, but I was assured that, given Liam's condition when he was first born, he was progressing as he expected. I complained that I believed Liam's health had actually deteriorated since his birth. The paediatrician confirmed that I was correct, but that this again was quite normal. Premature babies usually do get worse before they get better.

Instead of just being told that he would be better 'soon' or 'in a few days', I was given some more realistic goals and targets by which to measure my son's progress. He thought it would be a week to ten days from birth before Liam was breathing unaided. After that, we would have to tackle the problem of feeding. Premature babies have often not yet acquired the sucking reflex. It could be up to his original due date before Liam was allowed home, but the paediatrician hoped that maybe he would be home some time in the period between Christmas and New Year. This I could live with. We were talking about 'when' Liam would be better and I just had to make it through the few weeks until then.

My next concern was not to be discharged without Liam. I couldn't bear the thought of going home without him. I'd taken Stephen to hospital in Sheffield and travelled home alone. I didn't want that to happen with Liam. I was told I would have to talk to the hospital administration staff. If I was progressing well, I would normally be discharged after around five days. However, everyone acknowledged that this was hardly a normal situation. Once home, I'd be besieged by the media while my son was in a hospital some 20 miles away. How would I fit in expressing milk, dealing with the mob and visiting my son?

I was told that I could have Liam moved to Bassetlaw Hospital once he was out of Intensive Care, but I didn't want that to happen. First, it represented an unnecessary potential breach of confidentiality about his health, and second, I trusted the Jessop Hospital staff to take care of him. I wanted those same people to see him well enough to go home. I thought it important for Liam to have continuity of care and also for me not to have to start new relationships with those looking after him. I'd built up a special rapport with one of the nursing sisters on nights, as I particularly liked visiting Liam during the night when the ward was quiet and peaceful. The nurses, and also the paediatrician on duty, had more time to explain things to me at that time, Liam had his most wakeful period between midnight and 3 a.m., and I didn't have the problem of a continuing stream of visitors myself. I would hardly be able to visit in the dead of night if I was discharged, and that would be a great shame. I really felt that Liam and I were getting to know one another during my midnight vigils.

Fortunately, the hospital administration staff were sympathetic to my request to stay on the ward. I was lucky because the Jessop had so few patients in maternity at that time. It was no problem for me to remain in hospital, although everyone thought I might want to spend Christmas at home. I did, but not without Liam. I wanted to spend Christmas Day with my son, wherever that might be. We decided to tackle the problem of Christmas Day when it arose. We still had ten more days to go until Christmas Eve.

In the big outside world beyond the hospital cocoon, things were hotting up with the media. They were still baying to speak to 'Diane Blood'. It wasn't only me who was burning the candle at both ends, my parents were too. They were visiting me in the day and then trying to stave off the media when they left. My father also had an additional job. When I'd been admitted to hospital, my new bathroom, which I'd ordered when I first became pregnant, was still only partially complete. The job had turned out to be a complete nightmare. Everything that possibly could go wrong had done so. He was trying to sort it out and get it finished for when we came home. At that time, I didn't even have running water.

When my parents arrived that Monday, they told me that I really had to speak to the media. It seemed no one would be satisfied until they'd heard from me. Once it was over and done with, perhaps they'd leave us in peace and my parents could get some sleep at night. The offers for exclusive deals were still flooding in. In particular, they wanted the first photo of Liam, but I wouldn't allow his photograph to be printed whilst he was ill. I didn't want the world's first glimpse of my darling son to show him wired up to monitors, wearing nothing but an over-large nappy and a woolly hat to hold his tubes in place.

I had taken photographs myself but hadn't dared to have them developed. I was afraid the negatives or a few additional prints might get diverted to a newspaper somewhere between the processing laboratory and whoever went to pick them up on my behalf. I even sent my camera home at night with my parents for fear it would be stolen whilst I was asleep or away from my room. For this reason, I was totally reliant on Polaroid images of Liam. I had three of them Blu-tacked to my hospital locker. They weren't the best photos in the world, but they were all I had. In the absence of anything better, the media would have settled for them too, but they weren't on offer. I'd consider having a press conference, but there would be no photograph released.

I went to visit Liam again whilst I thought about our options. He didn't care, he just wanted to get by with the next breath. I stood longingly stroking the glass barrier of his incubator. The nursing sister asked if I wanted to hold him for a short while.

'Will he be all right?' I asked, 'I don't want to do anything that would harm him.'

'He'll be OK for just a quick cuddle. I've got to change his bedding anyway, so if you sit down and put a cushion on your knee, we'll lift him out, make sure none of his wires are tangled and then you can hold him whilst we change his sheet.'

I couldn't believe it. We were going to be allowed our first cuddle. I eagerly trotted over to the sink to wash my hands and arms, whilst someone went to fetch me a cushion and placed a chair, especially selected for its stability, in the small space between Liam's incubator and the ward door. I sat expectantly, arms poised facing upwards, resting on top of the cushion. Liam was placed, like precious china, in my waiting arms.

For a few seconds I was anxious, whilst the sister smoothed out the wires and traced each one back to its monitor. She checked they were all functioning correctly. I held my breath, then I exhaled, releasing my trepidation. My heart beat more slowly and a wave of calm engulfed our little corner of the room. I was completely wrapped up in the tiny little bundle of warmth enveloped next to my bare skin, beneath my dressing gown.

I held him close, my eyes fixed on the monitor displaying Liam's breathing, just in case I caused him any distress. The little bars of vertical red light normally danced around the 50 per cent mark, halfway up the monitor. If they fell too much below that, the machine would bleep and the nurses would have to increase the amount of oxygen Liam was given. If they increased to 90 per cent, the amount could be reduced. I was waiting for the dreaded bleep as the bars fell, but, on the contrary, the towers of red light stretched continually upwards. Liam's oxygen was reduced again and again. This boy needed his mum. He needed to be held and loved.

The nurses smiled, 'I think you've cracked it.'

'Can you stop awake 24 hours a day to cuddle him better?' another added, with a slight hint of laughter.

'Whatever it takes,' I replied.

I was aware that the sheet-changing exercise had been completed quite a while ago, but I was not pressed to hurry and return Liam to his incubator. He was obviously not in any distress, but I was concerned not to push my luck too far and so I asked the sister to put him back for me.

She lifted my responsibility tenderly from my arms. 'Good boy. Perhaps you can have another cuddle with Mum tomorrow.'

The incubator safely closed, I watched as Liam's breathing stabilised again. Sadly, his oxygen requirements increased, but not quite to the level they had been before our little cuddle.

I left Special Care relieved and content. It was the first time I'd noted any progress with Liam's health. I think the cuddle had done us both the world of good.

I returned to my room and told my parents I was ready to face the media.

CHAPTER 20

Going home

My parents quickly got to work arranging a conference in the hospital boardroom for later that afternoon. We weren't really prepared. It was a fire-fighting exercise. I didn't even have any daytime clothes at the hospital and there was no time to send anyone to fetch them.

My father thought I must be feeling better because I'd started to care about how I looked. I had no make-up either, but I asked him to get one of the female TV crew members to bring some with her. I also considered temporarily removing my 'sexy', white elastic, post-operative stockings. They help maintain good circulation and thus prevent blood clots. In the end, given our family history of thrombosis and the fact that they would be so incredibly difficult to put back on, I decided against it. Instead, I settled on a long white cotton nightgown which would cover my legs. Or rather, two long cotton night gowns, one on top of the other. When you stood against the light, each was transparent. I didn't wish to imitate Princess Diana's first photo call outside the nursery following her engagement to Prince Charles. She might have had the legs to look good despite her flimsy skirt and lack of undergarments. In these stockings, I certainly did not.

It was a long walk to the hospital boardroom, given that I had only recently dispensed with the wheelchair after the Caesarean. We went down in the elevator and then I gingerly made my way along the lengthy corridor, clutching Rudolf, a reindeer cuddly toy that my cousin had bought for Liam. The cameras were rolling. The lights were on. The flashes beamed, as one photographer after another called my name.

'Diane, this way.'

'Diane, smile.'

'Into this lens, please.'

'Diane. Could you lift the toy nearer to your face?'

'Thank you. That's lovely.'

'Diane, could you just stop there by the Christmas tree a moment?'

I stopped, posing by the brightly lit tree outside the boardroom door.

A few reporters began asking questions, 'What did you get Liam for Christmas?'

I misheard the question. The idea of me having had the chance to purchase a Christmas gift for my son was so bizarre that I'm sure I could have been forgiven. I actually thought I was being asked what I had got for Christmas.

'Liam,' I replied.

It wasn't until the reporter repeated my answer, in the tone of voice that implied I was completely ga-ga, that I realised my mistake. It was too late to go back and correct myself. I was already being bombarded with other questions. I halted my responses so that we could make our way into the boardroom. I wanted to give everyone a fair chance and, above all, I wanted to sit down. I was accompanied by all four of Liam's grandparents. I sat in the middle, placing Rudolf, the cuddly toy, on a ledge behind me. The journalists didn't like that. They wanted Rudolf on the table in front of me, so he was rapidly moved back to star position.

The reporters seemed to have two key routes of questioning. First, they wanted to know if I'd be trying for a baby brother or sister for my newborn son. I found this very strange. I thought we were here to talk about Liam. I'd only just had one baby and it was taking up all my time just thinking about him. I told them so and they seemed to accept this as a reasonable answer.

Second, they'd just rediscovered that I wouldn't be allowed to name Liam's father on his birth certificate and they thought we could start an effective campaign to get this ridiculous rule overturned. I agreed with them that it was rather stupid, but I didn't really want to go on about it at that moment in time. I thought it would be nice if that was all I had to worry about.

I told the journalists that Liam needed everyone's prayers, as he was still very ill. I felt much better for getting that one out in the open because I felt that everyone had been ignoring the fact that my poor little son was still in Intensive Care, battling away for breath.

As a pack, they were desperate for a photo. I explained that I wouldn't allow him to be photographed whilst he was in Special Care and I refused to hand over my precious Polaroids, which I said I needed to help me express milk. They had no alternative but to accept what I said. As individuals, many of the photographers and reporters sympathised with my uncooperative stance on the photos. They told me not to be pushed around and said that I should sell his photos to the highest bidder. They told me that they were worth a fortune and that they were all making stacks of money out of us, so why shouldn't we take a slice? Some reporters had also bought gifts for my son, not purchased by their employers, but from themselves and their families. I found this very touching.

The press conference finally over, I returned to my room, exhausted, relieved and a little emotional. Mum and Dad went home and I began to cry. I just wanted Liam to get better. I was sure now the public would understand he wasn't well and pray for his recovery. Between my sobs, I also began to say a little prayer for him. I was interrupted by a nurse. She entered the room clutching one of my small jars of expressed milk from the fridge. She held the few drops up to the light so we could both examine the meagre contents. Do you have any more milk expressed? The nurses on Special Care are asking for milk for Liam.

I jumped up. 'Is he taking milk? He couldn't digest it before. Is he improving?'

The nurse didn't know. All she knew was that they were asking for more milk.

I was ecstatic. I had no more supplies already expressed, but I quickly got on with the job of producing some more. If my son was getting better, I could do anything. 'How much milk does he need?'

'As much as you can manage.'

I expected it to flow out, but sadly my breasts didn't quite live up to my expectations. I produced a reasonable amount, but it was a bit of a trade-off between time and quantity. They needed the milk quickly and also I was eager to go and see my son and ask about his sudden progression to milk.

They were waiting for my arrival on Special Care. They took the little bottle of milk I was clutching and quickly poured it down the feeding tube into Liam's stomach. There wasn't quite enough, so they had to top up with formula.

Once the milk was administered, I had time to ask about this new development. I was sure it was a good sign. I was praying for Liam's recovery, I'd asked the public to pray for him and now he needed milk. The news wasn't quite so good. Some essential vitamins and minerals were missing from Liam's stomach contents. They didn't have the correct fluid to replenish these and didn't have time to get it. They thought they'd try him on milk, which would serve the same purpose. Unfortunately, however, Liam's little stomach couldn't take the new white stuff and he was sick. All my hard work with the expressing was thrown back in just a few minutes. I clung to the hope that maybe he'd extracted some goodness from it in the short time it had remained in his tummy.

The following morning brought more cards and kind wishes from the public. They had been listening. They hoped that my son would get better soon and I drew real strength from some of the letters I received. People told me how they'd felt when their children were in Special Care and how those same children had grown up to be strapping lads and lasses, with no hint of their early problems.

Liam finally showed signs of improvement. When he began to get better, it happened quite quickly. He came off CPAP in the early hours of the morning on Thursday, 17 December. Little pipes still blew oxygen into the bottom of his nose to gently assist his breathing, but he had fewer pipes and he was more reliant on his own resources. We could also dispense with the woolly hat, which I was pleased about. Liam had such beautiful hair it had been a shame to cover it up. The paediatricians told me that he would probably have to go back on CPAP when he got tired with the new effort he was exerting. But my son didn't turn back. Once he came off CPAP, he stayed off for good. Unfortunately, he did have a new problem with jaundice. He had been borderline for a while, but now they had to treat him with the sun lamp. He looked like he was sunbathing, with his tiny goggles protecting his eyes and one arm lifted above his head. 'Just getting a tan on this side, Mum. Don't disturb me.'

The following evening when I went to visit him, I found him missing from his usual position by the door of Intensive Care. The sister who had been such a help to me on the night shifts was on again. She met me just inside the door of the baby unit.

'He's been promoted. He's in here.' She led me across the Special Care corridor to the High Dependency ward.

She had also moved wards, so she was still looking after my son, which I was grateful for. The High Dependency ward was so peaceful after the glare and alarms of Instensive Care. They tried to keep the lights dimmed at night so that the babies got used to the difference between night and day. In this ward there were just four babies, a few mobiles and toys, and a little lamp glowing away on the shelf.

This time was very special. I was less anxious about Liam's health and that evening, the sister took him out of his incubator, dressed him and put him in a cot. Dispensing with the glass barrier was, I felt, a huge step forward for our mother–son relationship. Liam had never liked the incubator. He tried to climb out of the port holes every time you opened them. I think he felt rather exposed with no clothes on and the sister said she thought he would feel more secure when he was wrapped up in a blanket. He did seem much happier and he turned to the smell of my milk.

The nurses joked that he could smell me whenever I came into Special Care because he was always quiet before I arrived, but he would cry the minute I came near the ward. The sound of a baby crying is beautiful when you have had to wait so long to hear it. Special Care wards are so quiet: the babies are too ill to make their voices heard.

The next battle was feeding. Gradually, over the next couple of days, my son was introduced to milk in steadily increasing quantities. I helped to feed him by pouring the milk down the tube into his tummy. I tried to supply enough breast milk, but he was on about 40 per cent formula to top up the quantity. They were aiming to space the feeds out until he could go two to three hours between each one. I would need this gap when I took him home. We also had to progress to breastfeeding.

Liam seemed eager to try this one. Whenever we cuddled, he would root out my nipple. He tried to latch on, but he put his tongue up to the roof of his mouth. With my nipple under his tongue, sucking was impossible and he would fall off. It was very frustrating. Thankfully, the sister suggested using a nipple shield just until he got used to putting his tongue down. It worked. Only a few sucks at first, but I finally managed to breastfeed my son. I was elated that he'd finally got some milk from me.

It was 20 December. Everyone was in the festive spirit. The only blot on the horizon was that the sister had heard a politician doing a radio interview in which she had said words to the effect that she thought my son should not have been born. The sister had been driving into work and couldn't believe how someone could say that about the tiny baby she was trying to nurse back to life. I couldn't believe that someone could say that about my beautiful, courageous son. He was trying so hard to get well.

The 21st of December, the longest night of the year, was the night everything finally came together. Liam finally breathed unaided for the first time. We weighed him: 5 lb 4 oz; measured his head circumference for the first time: 31.4 cm; and his length too: 48.5 cm.

In the dead of the night, helped by the sister, I gave him his first bath. Liam yelled his head off. I was nervous that I was upsetting him, but it was great to hear his lungs in full action. Finally, we learnt to breastfeed, without the aid of the nipple shield. It's a good job it was such a long night. We achieved such a lot together and it was a wonderful time.

I sat up with Liam right throughout the night, waiting for the paediatricians to do their rounds the following morning. The sister gave Liam a glowing report and, in view of the fact that we were not leaving the hospital just yet, Liam was allowed up onto the ward with me.

He went for his hearing test, which he passed, and then a nurse brought him to me on the ward. My visitors could finally come to see Liam and me both together, and I could show off just how precious and beautiful he was. I was very proud of him.

The chief occupation of the next few days was just being a mother and enjoying my son's company. The next most pressing job was to decide what to do about Liam's photos. I couldn't not release anything. I would be hounded from the moment I got out of the hospital and whoever managed to snap the first photo would take control of the market. They'd get all the money. They would probably sell to the *News of the World* (as their circulation figures usually mean they can afford to pay the most), cutting out all the other papers, and it might even be a horrendous photo.

I'm not an angel. I found the idea of easy wealth created by signing an exclusive deal with just one newspaper a rather tempting proposition. The money, of course, would go to Liam. I could use it to pay for his education. I could even almost buy the papers' sales pitch. Sign up with one and they'll protect you from the rest. But how could I choose which one? If I signed with the *Express*, it would be poor thanks to the readers of the *Mirror,* who'd given me so much support, and vice versa.

I felt a bit lost and exposed. There was a definite attraction to thinking that the editor of one paper would look after us and take care of everything. It was just that the nagging voice in the back of my head kept reminding me that Liam really had only me to protect his interests. At the end of the day, no one else qualified for the job. I couldn't hand over control to anyone else. My decision was made. I wanted Liam to have the copyright on his first photos and I wanted everyone to have the opportunity to print them. I'd organise a photo shoot myself, ask for a contract giving us copyright from the photographer and put them out to an agency to distribute and negotiate fees on a non-exclusive basis. Liam would then be paid a percentage royalty fee each time they appeared. He would get some money, but not as much as he could have.

I asked my father to call a Sheffield photographer called Andy Gallacher, whom I'd worked with in the past on advertising projects involving children. He was a good photographer, but, most important of all, I trusted him. This was difficult, considering what had happened with my wedding photos. As the wedding photographer owned the copyright, he was paid all the royalties generated by their publication. Neither I nor the Stephen Blood Baby Appeal ever received any of the proceeds.

At first, my father really didn't like the idea of trusting another photographer. I think he'd rather have gone with the newspaper editors, but once he'd spoken to Andy, he had to admit he seemed very organised and affable. To be honest, I'd almost run out of time. We were hoping that Liam and I might be able to go home for Christmas and I had to have photos in the can before we left the hospital. I didn't necessarily have to release them just yet, but they had to be there, ready and waiting, in case someone else managed to get a snap and started calling the shots about publication in the interim.

Going home

It was the afternoon before Christmas Eve. The advertising and photography industries tend to close early for Christmas and don't reopen until the New Year. Most people had already packed up and were well into the festive spirit.

Fortunately for me, Andy was still working and turned out to be both honourable and organised. The shoot was scheduled for the following morning. I'd arranged hundreds of photo shoots, but for this one my head just wasn't working properly. It was Andy who thought to hire the stylist and find one willing to work on Christmas Eve at such short notice. It was Andy who booked the necessary couriers and he also called the lab to request express processing and for it to stay open late on Christmas Eve. In a way, it was also Andy who worried about the cost. We just agreed not to fall out over money and to sort it all out later. I had to trust him because there wasn't time for him to keep coming back to me and ask if every little thing was OK, and he had to trust me not to see him out of pocket and to try and get his name mentioned when the photographs were printed. The only fee paid in advance was the princely sum of one pound, the price exchanged for the copyright.

I didn't enjoy the photo shoot. It was a lot to cope with. And these were people I knew. Goodness knows what I'd have been like with a bunch of strangers fussing around, positioning my precious baby. To get the kind of shots the publications would want, I had to hold Liam's face close to mine. This is quite unnatural with such a tiny baby. In reality, you'd hold them much lower. I had to have frequent rests because my arms were so strained holding him in such an awkward position. Basically, we just shot rolls of film until I'd had enough. We could really have done with some more, but we decided that if I didn't get pushed into releasing the photos before, we could do another shoot between Christmas and New Year at home and then maybe release them on New Year's Eve. It would be nice to have some photos at home, perhaps near the Christmas tree, as well as those taken at the hospital There's only so much you can take at one go and I was worried about Liam. I didn't want to disrupt him too much after he'd been so ill, not that he seemed to mind or particularly notice. He slept through most of the proceedings.

Relieved the photography session was over, I went back to my room (which was still crammed with cards and flowers) to get some rest. For the shoot we'd taken over the slightly larger, and much tidier, room next door. Cocooned inside the hospital, it was easy to forget it was almost Christmas. It looked like we weren't going to make it home for Christmas Day after all. When the paediatrician had been round to check on Liam in the morning, she'd been very concerned. At 5 lb 4 oz, he was still very tiny to be going home, but she had said this was all right. She was more concerned about his colour. He was still very jaundiced and she'd sent some blood to be tested. We were still waiting for the results.

Finally, the paediatrician arrived back with the news. Liam's jaundice wasn't as bad as it looked. We could go home so long as the community midwives kept an eye on it. It was just before 3 p.m. Professor Cooke heard that we were to be allowed home for Christmas and called to see us before we left. We took the opportunity to take a souvenir photo of us all together and said some fond goodbyes to all those who had helped us at the Jessop Hospital.

By the time Liam and I could leave hospital, it was much later in the day. We had to complete the discharge papers, pack my bags and gather up the cards, gifts and various mementos of the flowers and balloons. We left most of the flowers on the ward. I couldn't possibly have taken them all home. Finally, Liam was wrapped up in a hat and shawl and we were ready to face the outside world.

A nurse came with us to the door of the hospital, wheeling my precious little bundle in his cot. We stopped by the hospital Christmas tree, outside the boardroom, so I could take one last photo of Liam leaving the hospital. The cold beckoned from the outer door just opposite. We lifted Liam from his cot. My dad had already driven the car up to the door to wait for us.

It was dark outside and everything was strangely quiet. No fuss now. No waiting journalists. They'd all gone home to spend Christmas with their families. No voices of congratulations or dissent. Just my parents, myself, my son and a journey home. Almost four years earlier, I'd been forced to return home without my husband, leaving him behind at the hospital in Sheffield. This time, our son was safe and sound at my side. This was what it was all about. At the end of the day, it was just us: one small family in a very big world. Nothing particularly remarkable about us, but it was an incredible journey against almost impossible odds.

God gave an extra miracle that Christmas and the story cries out to be told. This is only the beginning.

CHAPTER 21

A new life together

Liam turned my little bungalow into a home for the first time. Someone had put my Christmas tree up for me. The tiny wooden crib I had so carefully chosen had been erected and placed next to my bed. The rooms were warm and welcoming, waiting for the new baby. Now my home was full of life. Lots of people came to visit. Since my husband's death, people had tended to expect me, as a single person with no ties, to go and visit them.

My mother stayed over initially. I was still recovering from the Caesarean and Liam was quite a handful. I'd been sent home with instructions to feed him every two hours until he gained more weight. That first Christmas Eve at home together, I placed him in his little crib and went straight to bed. At night I'd been told we could go three hours between feeds if he was asleep, but then I had to wake him. If he'd have slept for three-hour stretches that would have been great, but Liam hadn't read my instructions and had a completely different agenda. He'd demand to be fed every 20 minutes or so for a few hours and then, when he finally dropped off to a deep sleep, he'd refuse to wake after the allotted time. Before beginning the task of breastfeeding, I'd have to spend ages trying to coax him to suck. At first, I'd stroke his tiny cheeks. If that didn't work, I had to tweak his ears or flick his heels. In practice, this meant that a 20-minute feed turned into a 40-minute stretch. By eight o'clock in the morning, I was exhausted and very relieved if my mother was awake to take over. She obviously couldn't feed

Liam for me, but just knowing that I didn't have to listen or clock-watch for a few hours was a great relief.

On Christmas morning, a couple of hours' sleep was the best gift she could have given me, which was just as well, as no one had had time to actually go out and buy anything. Even the fridge was empty, so we gratefully accepted an invitation to go to my cousin Julie's for Christmas lunch. We wrapped Liam in his beautiful crocheted shawl and took him for his first outing. Optimistically, we also took his carrycot in the hope that he might sleep long enough for me to eat my meal. He didn't, but there was no shortage of people offering to give him a cuddle.

We stayed for the meal and a couple of photos, but then went more or less straight home. I was expecting the midwife to call. They are supposed to visit you on your first day at home, but she didn't come. I assumed it was just because it was Christmas Day, but when a midwife finally arrived on Boxing Day, she assured me that Christmas Day should have been no exception. Apparently, as I had been discharged from hospital so late on Christmas Eve, the paperwork hadn't been sorted and no one had registered that I was at home until the next day.

I had a few relaxed moments in our first couple of weeks at home. I was so proud when I took Liam for his first walk in the pram. Friends, neighbours and even total strangers, who saw us through their windows, rushed out to see us. I was a little embarrassed when Liam screamed all the way home, but at least everyone knew we were coming. My mother said she could hear us from the bottom of the street. It seemed a welcome, if not very peaceful, introduction to a new, more relaxed pace of life. I wish that it could have always been so. I enjoyed thinking solely about my little baby, but I had pressing concerns because of the number of requests for interviews and because I still hadn't released the photos.

I had delayed it as long as possible, but time was now running out. We organised another photo shoot with Andy and shot some video footage with Central TV on the understanding that they would pool it to everyone else. Both the still photos and the news footage were finally released on New Year's Eve.

I thought it would end there. The new year would herald a new start and the interest would cease, but it didn't. Researchers were calling us from all over the world. I had another request from the

Oprah Winfrey Show. I really don't know how they thought a woman with a small, fragile baby could travel all the way to the other side of the world to do an interview. In the end, I agreed to just two requests. The first was from *Breakfast with Frost*. It addresses serious political issues and I felt I owed them, as I'd been on their programme before. Most of the programme was scheduled to be an interview with the Prime Minister, but Liam didn't get to meet him, as I insisted we were filmed at home. The second was a short interview for a programme to celebrate the 21st birthday of Louise Brown, the first test-tube baby. It would discuss ethical issues in fertility treatments over the years and other people would be talking about my case in any event. In particular, Ruth Deech had been invited to comment, so I felt I needed to balance it out.

I learnt quite a lot from the producers of that programme. I had taken so much flak over the years about how my child might feel about the unconventional circumstances of their birth, but these people had interviewed virtually every child born in ground-breaking and often controversial situations. They told me that if you asked them how they felt about the circumstances of their birth, they didn't know what to say, as it wasn't something they'd ever considered.

'It's a bit like asking how you feel about being English,' is how the producer put it. 'What is . . . is.'

After the immediate interview requests came the job of thanking all those who'd sent me cards and gifts. This was another daunting task because there were so many and everyone wanted a photo. I used the negatives from our photo shoot to get prints for those who'd given us special help and then printed postcards for the hundreds of others who'd written with their congratulations and encouragement. It took me about a month to do, snatching moments whenever Liam was asleep. It was difficult because it took so much time, but it was lovely, too, because it meant that I finally read all the letters. Not just those from Liam's birth, but the many hundreds more that I'd been sent during the court case as well. When I'd received many of them, I'd been too caught up in dealing with the case to really take them in or to respond properly at the time.

There couldn't have been a prouder mother in Europe. Liam was so handsome and I loved taking him out dressed in his tiny little knitted jackets, booties, hats and gloves. My mother-in-law,

Gill, had had many of them knitted for me, but many more came from members of the public. In particular, there was one little blue cardigan with red ladybird buttons. It was sent to me by an old lady and looked more like a doll's outfit than a baby's. Liam was so tiny that it was one of the few things I had which actually fitted him, so he wore it quite a lot.

The presents continued to arrive. Bettacare, a company who knew I worked for Clippasafe, sent me a bouncy seat and a car seat especially designed for premature babies. As Liam grew, I received bigger knitted cardigans from the public, a lovely cross-stitch picture for his bedroom wall and a playpen from a company named BabyDan.

I tried to forget about the court case, but sitting in my lounge drawer were the final conclusions and recommendations of the report by Professor Sheila McLean, 'Review of the common law provisions relating to the removal of gametes and of the consent provisions in the Human Fertilisation and Embryology Act 1990'. It had been published in the July before Liam had been born. I had skipped over its contents briefly, but then just stuffed it away to deal with later. I had until April to respond. It made pretty grim reading. Mostly it disagreed with my point of view, but it offered one slight ray of hope. Professor McLean had recommended that the law should perhaps be amended to allow deceased fathers to be named on the birth certificates of children conceived after their fathers' deaths, even though it should not be allowed to affect inheritance rights. The inheritance issue didn't concern me. The name on the birth certificate would have been great. However, new laws are rarely retrospective, so it looked like I may have helped others in the future, but it wouldn't benefit Liam.

This seemed most unfair and turned a situation which I had reluctantly accepted from the outset into something quite different. If a new law was passed which didn't include Liam, he would be one of only a handful of children to be singled out as being fatherless. New children conceived in the same circumstances would be treated differently and Liam would be discriminated against due solely to the timing of his birth. It even crossed my mind that, if I should ever try for a sibling for him, the new child could have their father named whilst Liam's birth certificate would remain unchanged. When I had gone to register him, I had been advised that I had to put a line through the spaces which were meant to record the paternal details. The normal explanation for this is that the father is unknown. I had tried desperately to get the registrar to accept an alternative which would distinguish Liam as a case apart. I wanted to write something along the lines of 'cannot be named due to the provisions of the Human Fertilisation and Embryology Act 1990', but this apparently wasn't an option. I couldn't even just leave it blank, which at least would have made me feel as though Steph hadn't been crossed out.

I responded fully to the Department of Health regarding the recommendations of the review, but in particular to the section on birth certificates. I pleaded that the new provision should be made retrospective. I also wrote an article for the *Sunday Telegraph* to appear on Mother's Day, shortly before the deadline for responses. The aim of the article was to highlight the issue and to try and get other members of the public to respond to the Department of Health as well. It was supposed to be a public consultation exercise, but I doubted the public even knew about it. How can you have an unbiased response when the only people in the know are those working in related professions?

It wasn't an easy decision to write about my family circumstances. Following my Court of Appeal victory, I was aware of a huge backlash from academic and medical circles regarding the amount of publicity we had generated. I didn't know what to do for the best. I couldn't take away the past, but I was worried about Liam's future welfare. Many self-professed experts seemed to want their say, so I decided to ask the only real expert I could think of. I rang Louise Brown to ask how she had been affected by the publicity and controversy surrounding her birth. Liam's birth, by comparison, had to be of minor significance. It was a private conversation, but the net result was that I decided to go ahead and write the article.

I do know that my *Telegraph* article prompted at least some response. A vicar sent me a copy of his letter telling how his own illegitimacy had caused him problems in his chosen profession and, most interestingly of all, I was contacted by Joanne Tarbuck. She was another mother whose child had been conceived after his father's death. Her son Jonathan had made the front page of the *Daily Mail* on 15 March 1997, the week after his birth and just a couple of weeks after I'd finally got permission to export Steph's sperm. I remembered reading and being questioned about her by the press at the time. She too wanted her late husband to be named on their child's birth certificate, so she responded to the Department of Health and we pledged to keep in touch.

After all this hard work, I really felt in need of a big party to celebrate and to thank all those who'd helped me along the way. Liam's baptism provided just such an opportunity. We erected a huge marquee on the back of my house. It covered the patio and most of the garden. It reminded me of the one that Steph and I had had on my parents' lawn for our wedding. Liam loved it. It provided hours of entertainment as he watched the big tent going up and, even though he was only a few months old, he was really quite excited by the activity.

The day was lovely. Liam was baptised at an Evangelical Church of England, which is just a stone's throw from our home. I had been taking Liam along to the family service since shortly after his birth, so we were known to the general congregation, as well as my invited guests. This made the day more special, as I really felt that everyone wanted to join in the celebration. We sang happy-clappy hymns and even the press photographers and reporters who were waiting outside said they felt a real sense of occasion. Some of my family came all the way from Ireland and some school friends who I hadn't seen for a very long time also joined us. The party went on long into the evening.

The following day, my birthday, was a real anticlimax. My parents were out with some of their friends who'd stayed overnight following the baptism. That's when I missed my husband. I wanted to relive the previous day and share the memories. The morning after our wedding, we'd talked endlessly about how wonderful it had all been, how pretty the marquee had been and how all the careful preparations had gone according to plan. The morning after Liam's baptism, it seemed the only thing to do was clear up the mess and go and buy the newspapers to see what they'd written about our special day.

I was finding my experiences as a mother quite different from that of my friends. This wasn't because I was single. Most of my friends had sole responsibility for their children during the day whilst their husbands worked, and a friend of mine has recently described to me how she too felt somewhat deflated after her daughter's baptism, notwithstanding the fact that she has a loving partner. No, the difference was because of the interest in our lives. The annual beautiful baby competition is quite a big event in our town. Everyone goes along to Woolworths to get their free photo taken. If I'd have gone, I'd have handed the photographer a free cheque to reproduce Liam's photo wherever he wished. For the same reason, I couldn't have his portrait taken, and, for a few months at least, I dared not take my own snaps in to local stores to be developed, so I had none to show around.

I also found that everyone, including complete strangers, wanted to hold my baby. Once I let a shop assistant hold him for a few moments because it felt impolite to say no, but then I felt very uncomfortable. I marked her every move, in case she dropped or ran off with him. Eventually, I learnt to explain why I felt I couldn't keep handing him over and people understood, but it was quite a learning curve.

I also felt that people invaded my space. They felt they knew me quite well, so they stood much closer than they normally would have done. They reached out for my hand and touched both myself and Liam. I didn't know them so it felt unnatural to me and, at times, quite unnerving. All the same, I was grateful to know that people obviously felt such affection for us.

Victoria Beckham had had a little boy named Brooklyn just a few weeks after I'd had Liam. I'm a bit too old to have been a real fan of the Spice Girls, but I would have loved to meet her to compare notes on things my friends had no experience of. I probably wouldn't have fitted into her world either, but I wondered if she attended special celebrity post-natal groups or if, like me, she would have loved to turn up to her local clinic but daren't in case the comments she made were reported to the press, or for fear she might offend the other mothers. Everyone thinks that their baby is the most special in the whole world, so it is difficult when yours is paid more attention.

I almost did get to meet her on one occasion. Liam and I were invited to a special awards ceremony organised by a newspaper. Victoria Beckham had been invited, too, and we could share the room which had been set aside for changing and breastfeeding. It sounded rather a grand affair, with loads of really important people. It was to honour and thank ordinary members of the public who had done extraordinary deeds. I was really looking forward to going, but, a couple of days before the event, I came out in blisterylooking spots. Liam followed suit, which confirmed my worst fears. We'd both contracted chicken pox. The timing meant we'd obviously caught it at Liam's baptism.

It was an awful time. I was aware that I'd never had chicken pox as a child and had been asked when pregnant if there were any of the usual childhood diseases that I hadn't had. I'd mentioned chicken pox and was told that it could cause complications if caught during pregnancy. A jab was available but, like everything, it came with a slight risk. I decided not to bother, as I had come into contact with the infection before but never caught it. I was sure I must have been immune. I obviously hadn't been, so I was at least grateful I hadn't caught it earlier.

For adults, chicken pox can be quite serious. I actually had a cousin who'd died from the complications it caused. He left behind a widow and two small children. I can remember Steph entertaining his children at some family gathering shortly after my cousin's death. Everyone else was sitting around talking and relaxing, whilst Steph crawled around with the kids under the table, playing house. I can remember quite clearly thinking how lucky I was that my children would have such a wonderful father and how unfortunate my late cousin's wife was that she no longer had anyone to help her.

As for myself, I wasn't exactly at death's door with the chicken pox, but I was extremely ill. I was also very worried about Liam. His tiny body was absolutely covered in red, angry-looking spots. There was hardly a gap between them. He wasn't quite five months old and, given that he had been a month premature in the first place, he was still very young to be fighting a disease. To make matters worse, I could no longer breastfeed, as my breasts were covered in weeping sores. I had enjoyed breastfeeding and didn't want to stop just yet, so, whilst trying to coax Liam to drink from a bottle, I still expressed milk to maintain my supply. It was hard work and I found sterilising the bottles a real chore, but, as always, my mum helped.

Thankfully, we both recovered with just a few minor scars to show for the experience, and life became easier and more relaxed. I really began to enjoy being a 'normal' mother. The press still called regularly, but I no longer feared that they would be lurking in the bushes. I once came home to find a reporter sitting on my drive. He'd driven all the way from Manchester for a comment about some new development in fertility ethics. I said I didn't want to comment. He understood and cheerfully set off back again without making too much fuss. An incredibly wasteful journey, I thought, but at least I felt I'd developed a reasonable relationship with the reporters. He'd come to my home because his bosses had asked him to, but he understood my reasons for not wanting to get involved.

I kept pretty much out of the public light until the autumn, when I agreed to speak at a fashion show during London Fashion Week. It was to help raise money for the Meningitis Trust, a charity obviously very dear to my heart due to the illness my husband had suffered. Lorraine Kelly was the main presenter. She was lovely, a terribly maternal figure, who enjoyed giving Liam a cuddle. The Calendar Girls, from the Women's Institute, were there too. This time they were modelling clothes, instead of taking them off. Lorraine Kelly took Liam into the next room to show him round. I must admit, I still hadn't got used to people walking off with him, even if it was Lorraine Kelly.

What was also remarkable about the fashion show was that a woman in the audience was considering posthumous conception. Unlike myself, she had no legal obstacles to overcome, but she had travelled down to speak to me and learn what she could from my experience. It seemed to me that all the counselling that was virtually forced upon these people must be failing miserably to provide the information required, due to lack of any real experience.

Christmas 1999 was just the best ever. It was soon to be the new millennium and Liam was old enough to appreciate the excitement. I loved taking him to see Father Christmas and buying gifts for him. He was in his bath one night when, from the bottom of the road, I heard the cheerful peal of carols, blurting from a loudspeaker. It was the Worksop Round Table. Each year, ever since I was a little girl, they go round all the streets at Christmas. Santa in his sleigh is pulled slowly along by a car. They stop wherever children come to greet them and Santa hands out sweeties. They had come up our road the Christmas before Steph's death. There were no children living on our street at the time, so Steph and I were the only people to go out.

'What would you like for Christmas?' we had been asked.

The National Lottery had just started and was still generating much excitement, so, despite the ridiculous odds against it, we replied that we'd like to win the lottery.

'I'll see what I can do,' joked Father Christmas, 'but you must share it with me.'

This year I felt I *had* won the lottery. The odds that my son would be born must have been even slimmer than the chance of winning all that money. Liam was the best gift I could have had.

I whisked him out of the bath and quickly wrapped him up in towels and a dressing gown. We sat on the front wall, awaiting the arrival of Father Christmas. Some neighbours came to join us when they saw that Liam was outside. Tears were streaming down my face because I was so happy. I wanted to say to Father Christmas, 'Look, we did win. Isn't it wonderful?' Of course, I didn't because he'd have wondered what on earth I was talking about. He did recognise us, though, and I think he shared a little of the wonder of Liam's birth.

Christmas passed and soon it was New Year's Eve: the millennium. I couldn't really go out because of Liam so I put him to sleep in his cot as normal and my parents came up to watch television and to see the New Year in with me. I cheerfully pranced around my home, videoing things that in years to come would remind Liam and myself of the momentous occasion. I repeatedly played Cliff Richard's 'Millennium Prayer' as the soundtrack to my filming, but always turned it back to the beginning before it reached the 'B' tune of the CD.

At midnight, the crack and spluttering of fireworks woke Liam up, so I lifted him out of his cot to show him the pretty colours twinkling through the windows. He loved it and bounced up and down in my arms as he reached out to try and catch the falling sparks. I really felt we were able to enjoy the moment together. My parents then went home, Liam went back to his cot and I was left alone, the 'Millennium Prayer' still in the CD player.

The millennium was a moment Steph and I had often talked about. We had assumed we'd both be there, probably sharing it with our family.

'Where are you now, Steph? Can you see us?'

Cliff Richard's version of The Lord's Prayer resonated around the room. I began to sing along and then to really offer up my words in prayer.

'Thy will be done on earth as in heaven . . .'

A few more sobs.

'Deliver us from evil for thine is the kingdom, the power and the glory.'

I stopped singing at the end of these familiar words. Cliff Richard sang another verse of his own whilst I continued to pray.

'Please, God, please give Steph a hug for me. Can he see his son? Does he know how beautiful he is? Does he know what I have been through?'

I cried my heart out and the CD continued onto the 'B' tune for the first time. Gradually, the words sifted through my tears into my consciousness. I could hardly believe what I was hearing. The song began:

> Like a dream my life has gone past me
> Taken so soon, but love burns so true.

I tried to stop crying in order to listen, as I realised that the words might be answering my prayer, but the tears still tumbled down my cheeks.

> Love never ending that shines like the stars in the sky

I had mentioned the stars in the sky in the poem I had written for Steph's epitaph. Perhaps this really was meant for me.

> And I sing, but so few can hear me
> Words from the heart to set your souls free.

I was no longer bound by the restrictions imposed by the HFEA and the subsequent battle. If only I could be sure that Steph had seen and knew that I had fulfilled his wish . . .

> Time has no distance deep in love . . .

This message really had to be for me. Apart from being a specific answer to the prayer I had just uttered, it was also a reference to my final message for Steph, written on the sundial that was his gravestone. At the time I had written it, my grief was so raw that I felt as though it would be an eternity before we were together again.

The glow of dawn could not compare
To the radiance of your smile
A midsummer's noon has not the warmth
Of the love we shared a while
And when the stars fill dark blue skies
Without the depth or brightness of your eyes
We mark the passage of another day
'Til we meet again . . .
I hope and pray.

Today, at the dawn of the new millennium, I was hoping and praying that Steph could be with us, and at that moment I felt that time and distance melted away through the words of the song still playing on my CD player.

Know everything goes
Everyone knows there's something beyond us
There is a light, believe me
Time turns into dust
Cry if you must
But love is the answer
Bringing two worlds together

Who can see the secrets that bind us?
Back to the earth 'til love burns so true
Eyes of compassion and the tears of a deepening heart

I have seen the pain of a cruel world
And reached out a hand for suffering to ease
Bringing some comfort to the tears

Somehow I felt that Steph had seen what I'd been through, and I realised that in my darkest moments I had felt his hand to ease my suffering. I felt his presence now, as I had felt it the night I prayed for someone to hold me.

Finally, there was a reference to the 'mountain of flowers' that there had been at Steph's funeral and the song ended with a repetition of its most poignant message:

Cry if you must
But love is the answer
Bringing two worlds together
Into one

Bringing two worlds together
Into one.

Love had brought our two worlds together to create one beautiful
little boy named Liam. I looked into Liam's eyes. His long, dark
lashes coming halfway down his cheeks just like his father's. By the
time the song finished, I knew that Steph had shared the
millennium with us. He had seen his wonderful son and I believe
that, whilst he is not omnipresent, he is there and will always be
there whenever he is thought of with love.

The power of this answered prayer made me feel as though I had
just been zapped by lightning. The thunderbolt didn't strike until
much later. When I finally contacted Craig Pruess, the lyricist of
the song, to seek permission to refer to its words in this book, I
learnt that it had been written as the result of a prophetic message.
A lady named Jennifer Lawrence rang him. She played out the
melody on a piano and told him that she had been told that he
should write the words, that the song would be sung by Cliff
Richard, it would be number one in the charts and would convey
deep meaning. It was written in 1998, the year Liam was conceived
and born. The words came to Craig Pruess in one sudden flash of
inspiration. He was driving along in his car, but had to pull over in
order to write them down. He told me that his idea was to write
the song as though it was Princess Diana speaking from the other
side, but to me, at that moment, it was my husband. More than
that: it was God's answer to the questions that I had asked.

CHAPTER 22

Paternity pursuit

At first, I had thought that I didn't have the stamina to try for a sibling for Liam. Of course, I hoped I wouldn't face any medical or legal opposition if I wished to try for another child using my late husband's sperm, but there was still the uncertainty of the actual treatment's success, not to mention the pregnancy and birth itself. I'd had my fair share of problems along the way with the last one and I didn't immediately fancy a repeat performance.

Still, from around autumn 1999, there commenced a growing voice in the back of my head reminding me that I didn't really wish Liam to grow up alone. We were such a small family. A brother or sister would make us feel more complete. When Steph was alive, we'd always talked of having more than one child. Steph thought the world of his two sisters and felt it was much better to be raised with siblings. As an only child, he had feared that I might feel differently, but I agreed. Circumstances permitting, we had settled on at least two, maybe three, children.

I didn't feel pressured by this. With him not being around to share the work and responsibility of being a parent, I'm sure that Steph would have understood if I'd stopped after Liam. The decision was for myself, Liam and the potential new child, not for my husband who was no longer here. By the New Year, my mind was made up. I was going to try again. Sadly, my body was not quite so willing and becoming pregnant for a second time proved difficult.

Meanwhile, the birth certificate issue was becoming more heated. I corresponded regularly with my lawyers regarding my options, while the press speculated on an imminent announcement following the report by Professor Sheila McLean. They predicted that the Government would agree to bring about legislation to allow deceased fathers to be named on birth certificates in cases such as ours but that it would not be made retrospective.

My QC from my first court case, Lord Lester, thought that I should seek legal remedy from the Court of Human Rights in Strasbourg. Lord Lester would be prepared to work on a no win, no fee basis. He was certain that my other lawyers would too, and, in Strasbourg, I couldn't get costs awarded against me if I lost. The problem with waiting was that the Human Rights Act 1998 was due to be introduced in October 2000. That might provide a domestic remedy, which would ultimately be quicker; but if I lost, then I'd be liable for the other side's costs. I knew from my first court experience that these could be roughly estimated at around £30,000, if I didn't take the case to appeal. We prepared the papers for Strasbourg and, in the spirit of the relatively recent 'cards on the table' approach to litigating, we submitted our draft complaint to the European Court of Human Rights to the Secretary of State for Health on 21 June 2000 before taking any further steps. This open approach was a sensible measure designed to help free up the courts by avoiding unnecessarily wasting court time. It had been introduced before my appeal and, for domestic courts, now formed part of the new CPR (Civil Procedure Rules) initiated by Lord Woolf when he was Master of the Rolls. He had just become Lord Chief Justice a couple of weeks earlier.

The rumours emanating from the Department of Health suddenly changed. It looked likely that the new law would be made retrospective after all. In any event, we were assured that an announcement would be made very soon, so we held off and held off, in the hope that all would be made clear before our October deadline for litigation in Strasbourg.

Finally, the announcement came on 25 August 2000. The Department of Health issued a press release confirming the Government's intentions to bring forward new legislation that would give me exactly what I had been asking for: my late husband's name on Liam's birth certificate. In addition, they would also change the law to allow sperm or eggs to be stored where consent hadn't been given but the person was likely to recover and might later express what is to be done with them. This was expected to mainly benefit a small group of children who undergo treatment for cancer but are too immature to understand and therefore give proper informed consent.

Whilst I feel this is a good thing in principle, in practice I think that, in my view, it doesn't go far enough, and may open up a can of worms. I have nightmares about people rushing to court in the middle of the night, arguing about best interests and whether someone is likely to recover or not. As regards children, testicular and ovarian tissue is already outside the remit of the Human Fertilisation and Embryology Act 1990, so may be and has been taken and stored in the child's best interests. For this law to be of benefit, the child would have to be mature enough to produce sperm or eggs, but not to have a clear understanding about their reproductive future. Whilst I'm sure that this does apply to some children, I would hope that the doctors do not set their standards too high with regard to satisfying themselves that the children fully understand.

I hoped that the two laws wouldn't be bundled together in one act, as I could see so many problems with the latter that I feared it would impede the progress of the birth certificate issue. I was assured that this would not be the case. To be honest, as no one is championing the case for limited storage without consent, unless it is part of a complete overhaul of the 1990 Act, I doubt it will ever happen.

The Government seem to sideline issues first by ordering lengthy consultations, then taking ages to make recommendations and finally hoping that everyone has forgotten about it all before they kick it out to the long grass, never to be seen or heard of again. This, I feared, is what they planned to do with my birth certificate promise. I wasn't about to let that happen. The press asked for comments, so I gave them. They asked why it was important, which seemed blatantly obvious to me. A birth certificate should be the truth. It was also important to my late husband's family and myself that they were given due recognition for their biological ties and that my son shouldn't be discriminated against due to the circumstances of his birth. If he ever got married, imagine how he and his bride would feel, leaving his paternal details blank on the marriage licence.

At this point, I felt that I would rather get this through by keeping it on the public agenda than by going to court again, if I could at all help it. The threatened action before Strasbourg was dropped in the light of the Government's new proposals. I was confident that it would all be sorted out very soon and cheerfully got on with the rest of my life, which was mostly idyllic and pretty care-free.

My biggest worry at the time was Liam's MMR (measles mumps and rubella) jab. My husband died of an infectious disease and I desperately wished there had been a vaccination to prevent it. However, like most mothers, I was still worried about the possible complications of the MMR that were being reported in the press and wondered if single vaccines would be better. Unlike most mothers, I also had a son who was allergic to egg. The MMR vaccine is prepared in egg, making him even more vulnerable to risk. Throughout the trials of the initial court case, I'd come into contact with many doctors throughout the world, so I now emailed them all, asking for their view on the safety of the MMR. They were all very pro-MMR and many seemed almost personally affronted that I should even question if it was right for my son. I rather felt that I was being labelled a paranoid mother with an over-precious son.

In the end, it was a mother from JABS (an acronym for Justice Awareness and Basic Support), who believed her own sons had been vaccine-damaged, that led me to the information I required to make up my own mind and not feel pressured. What I discovered was that, whilst the measles and rubella parts of the vaccination were available as single vaccines from the same source as those supplying them for the MMR, the mumps component was not. The strain that it covered was not that most prevalent in the UK. I went with the MMR because it had been used more widely than the single vaccines. It was rather a case of 'better the devil you know'. I decided that Liam should have the MMR and, thankfully, he had no problems afterwards.

The date of 1 October 2000 saw the introduction of the new domestic human rights law. Once again, the media wanted my comments. *Sky News* hurried round to film me on my back lawn and the telephone rang incessantly.

I felt strongly in favour of the new law and was in a position to know more than most, as I had attended the debate about it in the

House of Lords the night before my court victory and Lord Lester, my QC, had been the driving force behind it for the last 30 or so years. Also, I had felt frustrated that human rights arguments couldn't be properly addressed during my court case to fight for the right to try for my late husband's child. I don't know if they would have helped, but it would have made me feel more comfortable that all avenues had been explored.

It seemed to me that the Human Rights Act 1998 didn't actually bestow any new rights in itself. The rights it gave were already ensured by the European Convention on Human Rights, if you wanted to take the matter all the way to Strasbourg. It simply meant that they were more practical to pursue in terms of time and money. With my own case, this had been very important. It never made any sense to me that arguments which could have been easily dealt with alongside everything else in the domestic courtroom demanded a separate hearing with new judges who would have to start again from the beginning to understand the whole picture.

The downside of the new law was that it now meant that if I should need to litigate over Liam's birth certificate, costs would be awarded against me if I lost. Thankfully, at this point in time, I didn't believe that would be necessary. The Department of Health confirmed that I could tell *Sky News* in my human rights interview that they planned to bring in the new birth certificate law in the next parliamentary session.

As it was a Government proposal, I had assumed that it would be brought forward as Government legislation, meaning that it would be guaranteed parliamentary time. I was wrong. It was left to be taken up as a Private Member's Bill. Members of the House of Lords can introduce those at any time, whilst Members of Parliament from the House of Commons need to win a ballot, which is held at the beginning of each parliamentary term. The disadvantage with Private Member's Bills is that they are subject to time constraints and do not have the full force of the Government behind them.

To be honest, it seemed that the Government's promise to legislate didn't mean a lot. It had always been open to me to lobby Peers or Members of Parliament to take up the Bill themselves, but, following my experience with Lord Winston's Private Member's Bill in December 1996, this struck me as a complete waste of time. I could only hope that things were going on behind the scenes that would do more to secure this Bill's success if it was chosen from a Government handout list by someone that the Government was happy with.

All I could do was sit and wait. On 11 January 2001, I heard that Tony Clarke, MP for Northampton South, had taken on the Bill. This would be confirmed on the 16th. The only problem was that he had come 14th in the ballot. Those who had come higher up would have their Bills heard first. With a general election rumoured for May, it was going to be tough. Tony Clarke seemed quite optimistic, however, so I felt that I should support him fully and not allow my fears to put a damper on the proceedings.

The second reading was set for 23 March, which encouraged me, as it should have been a couple of weeks after that but had been pulled forward. I decided to do an interview about it for the *Daily Mail*, timed for the Saturday before the debate. Although I had some reservations about this, both myself and Tony Clarke felt we stood a better chance if the media were watching and reporting events.

Both my family and Joanne Tarbuck's family attended the debate in the House of Commons. The cameras followed our every move. There were supposed to only be a couple of Bills before ours, but unexpectedly the Government chose that day to announce an enquiry into the *Marchioness* disaster. This pushed everything back. The session ended at 2.30 p.m. If we didn't get our Bill read before then, we'd be back in the queue waiting for another date and the Bill would run out of time before the election. For Tony Clarke's Bill to make it, absolutely everything had to go according to plan.

We went into Westminster, but not immediately into the chamber because we had the children with us and they would have become irritable. Instead, we sat outside, watching events on the television, whilst Liam and Joanne's son Jonathan played together, blissfully ignorant of the mounting tension.

Tony Clarke came to give us regular updates. It was clear that a lot of negotiations were going on behind the scenes. People bargained for time and talks were held with anyone who wished to oppose the Bill. This is necessary in order to avoid wasting parliamentary time. It appeared that Eric Forth, MP for Bromley and Chislehurst, may be a bit of a problem. He didn't like Private Member's Bills that should really have been Government Bills and he had got himself a bit of a name as a serial Bill-buster. I prayed he'd let ours through. We bit our nails and watched the clock.

At ten to two, Tony Clarke made it onto the debating floor and we hurried into the public gallery to watch. To start with, all went swimmingly whilst our supporters said their piece, but then Eric Forth stood up and we all held our breath. At 2.20 p.m., Eric Forth was still on his feet and showing no signs of abating.

'Sit down, please shut up,' I urged beneath my breath, as I edged further and further towards the front of my seat.

Eric Forth was handed a small slip of paper, which he read whilst still in mid-flow. Miraculously and totally unexpectedly, he suddenly drew his speech to a rapid conclusion and sat down. Tony Clarke read the Bill for a second time. We made it through with only minutes to spare.

I didn't go to the next stage, which was the Committee. At that point, I didn't know the public were allowed to attend. It was held on 25 April, a Wednesday. I was told that Wednesdays were normally reserved for Government Bills only, so I believed the Government had made space for it and I felt heartened that they must be helping it along. *The Guardian* ran an article on their legal page the day before the debate and I was beginning to feel quite buoyant about the whole thing. I was assured that we only had to get it through the Commons. If it passed all its stages there, when the election was called it could go into what they called the 'wash-up'. This is basically when an agreement is reached to finish off all business which is uncontroversial and has made it through the majority of its parliamentary passage. I couldn't see anything remotely controversial about our birth certificate Bill, so I didn't think anyone else would either. I was about to be proved wrong.

Dr Evan Harris, Liberal Democrat MP for Oxford West and Abingdon, was one of the Bill's sponsors, so the last thing anyone expected was for him to suddenly throw a spanner in the works. He tabled lots of amendments for the Committee and appeared to have a massive problem with my case in particular. Anything he did or said seemed designed to prevent the Bill from applying to Liam. I couldn't understand this and demanded to know why he had made what seemed to be a handbrake turn. Nothing had been mentioned before and I had been led to believe there were no problems.

I was told by both Tony Clarke and the Department of Health that Ruth Deech had called Dr Evan Harris, who was her MP, the night before the Committee stage. She had expressed her very real concerns and these had led to his change of heart. Obviously, I wasn't party to the conversation between Ruth Deech and Dr Evan Harris, so I do not know the specific fears she imparted, but I presume from Evan Harris's amendments that she felt the Bill diluted the importance of the quality of consent. For instance, if there was no written confirmation that my husband wanted me to have our child after his death, then equally one couldn't be sure that he'd want to be named as a father on that child's birth certificate once it was born. I will never know the whole truth about the conversation which allegedly took place, but I was deeply wounded that my past court case seemed to be coming back to haunt Liam's future. I tried to get my supporters involved, but it was all too late. Opinions had been formed.

The Bill just scraped through the Committee stage, with no ground given that would block the Bill applying to Liam, and I was still assured it had every chance of success. It seemed unlikely that one of the Bill's sponsors would ultimately block its passage, once he saw that it could not be changed to exclude my son. I was sure that he would be told of my threat to litigate and, in any event, as long as the media were watching events, it was a possibility the Government couldn't allow to happen. We all knew there would be a public outcry.

The third reading was squeezed in for the following week, 27 April. Time was running out before a May election. At the eleventh hour, I decided to shoot down to London with my dad, so I could be there to give comments and also to lobby Dr Evan Harris. He was still trying to alter the Bill to exclude cases where the initial storage of the sperm had been unlawful. Even though in our case the HFEA had originally given permission for storage, this was intended to apply to Liam. Tony Clarke was already trying to get him to change his mind, but I felt that I too needed to be an advocate for my son. Even if the treatment leading to his birth had been totally illegal (which it certainly wasn't), it was nothing to do with Liam. Why should he be penalised?

The day was very tense, not only because of the drama with Dr Evan Harris but also because the High Hedges Bill, which was being debated before ours, went on for much longer than expected. Again, we had until only 2.30 p.m. for our Bill to be debated and read for a third time.

Time was marching on. I still hadn't managed to speak to Dr Evan Harris, although I was assured that others were doing so, and the High Hedges Bill was proving very resilient. It was never going to pass its reading that day because there were too many amendments, but attempts to kill it off swiftly so we could get onto ours were in vain. On a couple of occasions, a vote was called. If fewer than 40 MPs were around to vote, this would cause the Bill to fail. On the first vote it just scraped through, but finally, on the second vote, at almost 2.20, it failed to achieve the required number of votes.

We had only 13 minutes left and I still didn't know if Dr Evan Harris was a problem. We hurried into the public gallery to watch. The policeman who ushered us in assured me that all was well. He'd had a message that Dr Evan Harris had agreed to remove his amendments on the grounds that perhaps they could have been worded better, and his fears were in relation to future cases and not those which already existed. Eric Forth had conveniently 'gone to the toilet' and everything looked to be on track.

Yvette Cooper, the minister responsible for the Bill, entered the chamber to give her support. She looked up from the floor, nodded and smiled at me. As Tony Clarke entered, he gave me the thumbs up. The policeman sitting at the end of my row in the gallery smiled and said, 'That's it, you've got it.'

Tony Clarke drew his speech to a close just in time for the 2.30 p.m. deadline and then the unthinkable happened. Tory MP for New Forest West, Desmond Swayne, stood at the despatch box and talked the Bill out of time. You could hear the gasp of disbelief from the floor. People threw their arms into the air as they realised his intention. Even the Speaker looked totally confused. I looked at my dad. I thought perhaps I might find some clue on his face to assure me that this wasn't happening, but it was. The end of business was called and I left in tears. All that work, all that emotion, all that time and money – for nothing. We were back to square one.

I desperately wanted to speak to Desmond Swayne. I needed to understand why he had done what he did, but he had vanished from my life as quickly and silently as he had appeared. The media wanted to know what I would say to him. I decided to say something so shocking that he would realise how much his actions had wounded me. I accused him of effectively calling my son 'a bastard'. Never in a million years did it truly enter my head that anyone would think that about Liam, but the comment symbolised the deep hurt that I felt. Also, I knew that if I was ever going to get to speak to Desmond Swayne, I had to make him sit up and take notice.

By Monday morning, I regretted saying something so undignified, but by Monday afternoon Desmond Swayne had asked *The Independent* for my contact details. We spoke on the phone. He wanted to make it totally clear that he had no problem with my son having his father's name on his birth certificate, but he was concerned about similar cases in the future. It seemed that Desmond Swayne didn't understand the Bill terribly well. It was very tightly focused on paternity once the child was born. He appeared to think that it covered or endorsed the removal or dilution of consent for treatment. I questioned why he had spoken from the despatch box, as though he was presenting the view on behalf of the Conservative Party, when I had been led to believe that the Bill had cross-party support. He assured me that he had acted as an individual on a matter on conscience. However, Tony Clarke later put on record in Hansard that he had made comments to others claiming that 'he had intervened under orders'. It seems there is some confusion over this.

I had heard from Tony Clarke that moves were still afoot to try and get the Human Fertilisation and Embryology (Deceased Fathers) Bill, as it was called, into the wash-up, despite its failed third reading. Desmond Swayne reassured me that this was the case and said that he would have a word with Liam Fox (Shadow Minister for Health) and that he would be supportive of the move if Tony Clarke could give him the various assurances he was looking for. Maybe it wasn't all over yet. The last day of business before Parliament closed for the election was 11 May. If Steph had been alive, it would have been our tenth wedding anniversary. It seemed rather apt that if the Bill was to make it, it would do so on that day.

A frantic week followed, with many phone calls and emails being exchanged. Tony Clarke worked extremely hard, but on 9 May I was told of the discussions on the wash-up. The Tory Lords felt our Bill should not be included. Even if they had not objected, Dr Evan Harris had been present to have his say in any event. Maybe I had been a little naive to hope for such an outcome, but we'd achieved the impossible before, so I couldn't hide the fact that I was bitterly disappointed.

Still, the Department of Health encouraged me to remain optimistic. They confirmed via email that they would be 'working hard to introduce the Bill again as soon as possible in a way likely to bring success'. From various conversations, I understood this to mean that it would be a stand-alone Government Bill brought forward early in the new session, providing, as everyone expected them to, that Labour won the general election.

I had also generated some interest with a lobby group, the Townswomen's Guild, who had asked me to speak at their National Council Meeting at the Royal Albert Hall. I would speak for a few minutes, then an opponent of the Bill would put in their two pennies' worth, and members would vote on whether to support it and lobby on our behalf. I wasn't worried about the vote because, in my mind, our cause was sensible and uncontroversial. Sadly, as far as the Townswomen's Guild went, that proved to be our downfall. They couldn't find anyone prepared to speak against me, so my contribution was also dropped. Without it, members couldn't vote, so they couldn't lobby on our behalf. I am led to believe by someone who attended the meeting at the Royal Albert Hall that an announcement was made saying that the Human Fertilisation and Embryology (Deceased Fathers) Bill was not included, as the Government had already committed to introducing it. This had been true since August 2000 and well before they asked me to participate, but it didn't necessarily mean we were any closer to seeing it become law. However, at the time, I thought we were nearing the end of the road.

I watched the election with interest, praying that my supporters would retain their seats. Tony Clarke increased his marginal hold on Northampton South, Labour had an easy victory and I believed that our birth certificate Bill would be on the statute books by the end of the summer.

CHAPTER 23

Joel's birth

It dawned on me gradually that all was not going to go according to plan. The parliamentary session, which I had been advised would be really short, ending late in the summer of 2001, was now planned to end around November 2002. Our birth certificate Bill disappeared totally from everyone's agenda. There was no Government Bill in sight, no new Private Member's Bill and no hope of anything else happening until the next term, which wasn't for another year and a half.

The prospect of litigating became very real. Joanne Tarbuck and I spent much time on the telephone discussing it. Having got this far, neither of us was prepared to give up, but I was very afraid of facing a courtroom again and I was especially afraid of losing and ending up with costs awarded against me. Joanne was probably entitled to legal aid, and her son Jonathan certainly was, so this wouldn't be a problem to her. The prospect of Joanne litigating on her own seemed very attractive to me. If she won, the law would be changed and Liam would probably be entitled to have his birth certificate changed too.

There were two problems with this plan. First, Joanne had written consent for the use of her late husband's sperm. I did not. This meant that, whilst unlikely, a distinction might be drawn between our two cases. Second, the media were more likely to report events if I was involved. We figured that the Government didn't really care if they lost a lot of money fighting the case. They were more likely to be afraid of losing face.

The solicitors agreed to act on my behalf on a conditional fee agreement, which meant I had only minimal expenditure, court fees and so on, unless we lost – in which case I would be liable for the other side's costs. Still, it was a huge financial risk for a single mother to contemplate. I enquired about the prospect of taking out insurance against losing, but the type of action meant that it would be ridiculously expensive, if indeed it was possible at all. In any event, I couldn't apply until after a leave hearing, by which time we'd already be well on the way to preparing our cases.

My solicitors thought that Liam might be entitled to legal aid. I wasn't sure, as I'd invested the money which he'd made from the photographs of his birth in his name, but, in any case, I didn't think I could handle the potential backlash for taking money from the state. When I had fought for the right to try for Liam in the first place, many people had complained that he would be 'another mouth for us to feed'. I had promised that I had no intention of being a drain on the public purse. If I was going to litigate, I had to face the risk myself. I was still trying for another child. That in itself might prove controversial enough. If I became pregnant, I didn't want to give anyone any other ammunition to throw at me.

The solicitors began working earnestly on our case, whilst Liam and I got on with our lives. I tried not to let it intrude. It was important, but not of the same magnitude as my first court case.

The summer began happily enough, but then I found a small lump in one of my breasts. I thought that maybe I was imagining it, so I asked my mum to take a look. No, she thought there was a lump too. I went to see my doctor. He agreed and referred me to the hospital. I was in turmoil. Attempts to get pregnant were put on hold and for the first time I became desperately afraid and aware of my own mortality. I wondered what I had done. How would Liam cope if I became ill, or worse, if I wasn't there for him at all?

On the positive side of things, I began to appreciate every second we spent together. It was only two weeks until the hospital appointment, but we packed so much into each day. I remember one particularly sunny day when we went for a picnic in our local park. Liam was two and a half, and very inquisitive. He was asking loads of questions, about the sky, the clouds, the birds. It made me realise just how beautiful everything was and how wonderful it was to share my knowledge and appreciation with Liam.

The day of the hospital appointment came. I would have liked my mum to go with me, but I needed her to look after Liam, so I went alone. I had a mammogram and was examined by a specialist. The lump turned out to be nothing, probably just a pulled muscle. I've never been so relieved in my life.

That particular scare over with, I made plans to continue and try for a sibling for Liam. I'd been having the most awful dreams. I'd wake up to discover all the doors and windows to my home open and all the contents gone. The same vision presented itself over and over again, yet it always seemed so very realistic. I think I was afraid that something was missing and I wanted to put it right.

I was about to send some emails to liaise with doctors in Belgium about my treatment when I heard on the radio that the World Trade Center had been struck by terrorists. A news bulletin sent to my email address put the initial death toll at six, plus the passengers on the planes, but the radio had made it sound rather more serious. Like everyone, I was shell-shocked and wondered what kind of a world we are bequeathing to our children. For a day or so, time stood still as we repeatedly watched the images of colliding planes and collapsing towers. Liam wanted to know what it was all about and I didn't know what to say. When something so awful happens it seems almost uncaring that life moves on, but it always does.

The day I realised that I was pregnant was a little over a month later. My mum, dad and Liam had accompanied me to Belgium. It was a glorious, sunshiny day, and Liam was playing with some young Muslim children. I had only just had the treatment the day before, but my breasts were tingling with life. We were at a play park. The template for a game of hopscotch was marked out on the floor and Liam wanted to know how to play. I didn't want to show him for fear that jumping up and down might somehow shake the baby out of my womb. Fortunately, the other children were on hand to demonstrate the game to him, whilst my mother and I sat trying to talk with their young mother. She spoke no English at all. I spoke only a few words of French, but we still managed to converse about our children. I was blissfully happy. Life was wonderful after all.

I returned home a couple of days later and then had to wait just over a week for the pregnancy test. This time I asked a different local fertility clinic to monitor my hormones and progress following treatment, so that I could report the results to Belgium. The sensation in my breasts became less marked and I wondered if, in fact, it had not been because I was pregnant, but because of some hormones or something that I had taken at the time. The feeling had been so strong initially that I felt there had to be some radical explanation.

There was. Unlike with Liam, the pregnancy test was a good, strong positive. All I had to do now was to wait three more weeks for the scan to confirm that all was well.

Liam, my mother and a couple of nurses packed into the small room to stare at the monitor. There was one big, healthy-looking embryo with a little white flashing light that I knew was its heart beating away. To the side of it was another embryo, much smaller with a fainter flicker of a heartbeat. Even so, it was still looking more viable than Liam had been at his first scan, when he hadn't even had a heartbeat at all. I could hardly believe I was pregnant with twins.

A whole range of emotions swept over me, I was astonished and delighted, but frightened too. The prospect of us becoming a family of four really thrilled me, but, following my birth experience with Liam, I was worried that it might put the pregnancy at risk in its later stages. Liam had been so ill due to his premature birth; I didn't want that to happen again.

The doctors advised me that I should have another scan in two weeks. All I could do was report my results to Belgium and wait until then. As time went on, I really began to hope the little one would make it. To be honest, I was sure that it would, because it had looked so much healthier than Liam had done at the same stage. I prayed for both my embryos, but it was not to be. The next scan confirmed that the smaller of the two had not developed further and we had lost the heartbeat. God gave me two embryos, one that would continue to be nutured in my womb while the other would be looked after by Steph in heaven. The doctor told me that I might experience some bleeding because of it. I could vividly remember bleeding during my last pregnancy and I feared that it might flush out the surviving embryo. I prayed that I wouldn't bleed and I never did.

As with my first pregnancy, I suffered with dreadful nausea, which went on morning, noon and night. Even so, Christmas 2001 was especially happy. It seemed that I had achieved almost everything I could wish for, and Liam was at a lovely age, when the joy of Christmas spills over onto all around.

My pregnancy was a huge secret, as I couldn't afford news of it to leak out. My solicitor, Richard Stein, was one of the very few who knew. He was pleased when I accepted the invitation to Leigh, Day's annual Christmas party, so that he could congratulate me in person. My mum stayed at home to look after Liam, while my father and I went to the party in London. It was a chance to relax, unwind and celebrate. I didn't know many people there, but it seemed that everyone knew me and about my court case.

One person I did know was Clare Dyer, legal correspondent for *The Guardian* and the journalist to whom I'd given my very first interview. She was very chatty and, now that the trauma of my court case was over, I found that I warmed to her much more than I had done previously. We talked about the coverage of my case and I jokingly told her how I'd almost run away after our first interview.

'Well, I see you're not pregnant again,' she quipped. 'Now, that really would be a story.'

I laughed and rapidly changed the subject. Phew, that had been close. Richard Stein was standing next to me. I shot him a conspiratorial glance to see if he thought I'd got away with it. Clare didn't suspect a thing. The flared skirt that I had so carefully chosen to hide my small bump must have been very convincing.

I didn't explain properly to Liam until quite late in the pregnancy that he was to have a baby brother or sister. Three year olds are not renowned for keeping their mouths shut and, if you tell one person, you may as well tell the whole world. I regret the lost few months of shared excitement, but it's hard to see how I could have done anything else in the circumstances.

When I finally did tell Liam, it was great. We spent ages poring over baby-name books. If it was a girl, I still planned to name her Shannon, as my husband and I had decided, so Liam and I concentrated on picking a name for a boy. He was very enthusiastic about it all and couldn't decide whether he wanted the baby to be a boy or a girl.

At five months pregnant, I realised I couldn't hide my good news any longer. Liam had been told and my growing bump was becoming hard to disguise. People had started asking my family if I was pregnant and I believed the local paper was only one step away from discovering the truth.

I announced my pregnancy to the Press Association news agency on Friday, 8 February. It's a shame I didn't feel it could wait any longer, as I had my 20-week scan booked for the following Monday. It would have made me feel more comfortable to be able to confirm that everything was going well, but I really thought that it was that close to being leaked. I knew from my previous experience, when I'd been pregnant with Liam, that the worst thing that could happen was for one newspaper to find out before the others when you were not prepared.

Even so, I was still unprepared for the interest that the news caused. It soon became apparent that I would have to call a press conference to deal with the number of enquiries. A local public house, The Ashley, helped us out by providing a small upstairs function room. Liam was fascinated by all the cameras and attention. I had vaguely considered not taking him along, but I feared the press would find him anyway. I would sooner have him with me than for my family to end up split up and trying to deal with separate situations on their own.

Liam loves new babies and probably thinks that news of their pending arrival is always heralded with such fuss. He still remembers the cameras and I hope that one day it will help him to comprehend the interest in his own birth.

It was a very tiring and long day for all of us. By teatime, we were still at The Ashley. My mum took Liam downstairs to try and get him some food, whilst I recorded the last couple of live television interviews for local news channels. Liam watched it on the television in the pub.

'Where's Mummy?' he suddenly asked.

My mum pointed to the television.

'No, not that Mummy,' Liam replied, 'the real one.'

I was very relieved when it was over and I could go and give him a hug.

The news of my pregnancy was reported on the front pages of seven out of the eight major national daily newspapers. It was really strange wandering around the supermarket the next day. Normally, lots of people speak to me, but that day no one said a thing. They all just kept looking at me as if I shouldn't be there. I felt like shouting, 'Yes, it is me. Liam's real mummy has to go shopping like everyone else.'

At the time, it made me feel quite isolated and I wondered if everyone disagreed with my choice to have a second child, but the congratulations soon came flooding in. With hindsight, I think it was just that they didn't immediately know how to approach the subject when they'd heard it on the news rather than being told in person.

The news of my second pregnancy again raised the profile of my attempts to change the law regarding Liam's birth certificate. It became more urgent to me because I wanted it to be introduced before the new child was born. It became more important because I wanted my children to be recognised as full brothers or brother and sister. If both of their fathers were truly unknown, then logic says that it couldn't possibly be the same man. I wanted their full blood ties properly acknowledged.

A letter before action had been faxed to the Secretary of State for Health from my solicitors the day before my Press Association announcement. We told him of my good news, mentioning its relevance to the question of my children's birth certificates. John Mann, the new local MP for Bassetlaw, heard that I was expecting another child from the television and news reports that followed, and he decided to table a question in the House of Commons for the next week. The response by Robin Cook, who at the time was Leader of the House, absolutely astounded me. He said that he was 'not sure that the Government would have it in mind to introduce legislation on such a difficult and sensitive point, on which there are different views'.

So what was Professor Sheila McLean's report all about and the Government's grand announcement that it would retrospectively change the law? Was it just a load of hot air?

The best Robin Cook felt able to offer was that, 'if possible', they would make sure that a Private Member's Bill on the subject 'would receive a fair hearing in the House', if one were introduced. I felt badly let down and as though I'd obviously been completely wasting my time since beginning my campaign to change the law three years earlier. John Mann spoke with Yvette Cooper afterwards, who offered to meet with me.

We met on 7 March 2002. The deadline for responding to my solicitor's letter had passed the week before, but we hadn't received a reply.

Present at the meeting were myself, my father, John Mann,

Yvette Cooper, an official from the Department of Health and their press officer. Yvette Cooper seemed charming and genuine. They gave me assurances that Robin Cook had probably just not read his brief on the birth certificate question and that they were still doing their best to progress the matter with urgency. I made it clear that I was looking for a Government Bill, as I no longer believed that Private Member's Bills were a serious attempt to resolve the issue.

They sympathised but could offer no concrete plans with regard to timing or form. They tried to persuade me that litigating would be a waste of time because, even if we won, we would be no better off than we were now. Parliamentary time still had to be found to bring forward the Bill, which they had promised to do anyway. I told them that this was not true, as, if the court gave a declaration of incompatibility with the Human Rights Act 1998, they could amend the law by statutory instrument. In other words, they could bypass most of the political process by just amending the law on paper and then getting a parliamentary stamp of approval at the end. They would need only a few minutes instead of many hours.

Yvette Cooper and the Department of Health didn't seem to think this was an option. I couldn't understand why, because the decision to invoke the power to amend by statutory instrument in such a case rests with the Minister concerned. It depends on whether he or she thinks the matter is urgent. This was obviously where we disagreed. In my view, it was no longer acceptable to keep stringing us along. I told them that we would litigate. I would sooner take my chances with the power of a court judgement behind us. It was a gamble because, if we lost, we could potentially lose the ground already gained, but at that point I believed the Government's promises were empty. I'd been waiting two years already since the Department of Health announcement that the Government would change the law and I had seen nothing for my patience. They'd found parliamentary time to discuss shortening the working hours in the Commons to make it more family friendly – an issue affecting their children. What about mine?

Joanne Tarbuck eagerly awaited my report of the meeting with Yvette Cooper. Like myself, she was disappointed that they'd been unable to give us a finite timescale and agreed with me that it was time to stop pussyfooting around. We waited for the official response to our solicitor's letter before action and then steps began to start legal proceedings.

It was very scary. The possibility of losing so much money was not easy to accept. At the end of the day, I was a single mother with less than four months to go before my second baby was due. Thanks to the terrorist strike on 11 September and the subsequent stock-market crash, I had lost a substantial portion of the money I had invested for Liam from the sale of the photos at his birth. I thought I had been sensible, taking financial advice to place it in stocks and shares as it was a long-term investment for his education. With hindsight, this had proved to be a costly mistake.

I considered again the possibility of seeing if Liam was eligible for legal aid. If he wasn't, then the new baby certainly would be, but if we only litigated on behalf of the children then we could potentially miss some arguments that could be put forward on my own behalf. Like my children, I too claimed rights under articles 8 and 14 of the Human Rights Act 1998: the right to respect for private and family life without undue interference from the state and the right to enjoy this freedom without discrimination. Also, on my behalf, we could explore article 12: the right to marry and found a family, as well as some points of EC law. If any of the litigants were not legally aided, then it became largely irrelevant whether the others were or not, as the cost for the case was almost the same irrespective of the number of people pursuing the claim. The one who wasn't legally aided would be responsible for virtually all the costs.

As with my first court case, I decided I could leave no stone unturned. The papers were prepared on behalf of Jonathan Tarbuck, myself, Liam and my second child. We waited for the birth to insert the name. No one from my family applied for legal aid; Jonathan Tarbuck did. If we lost, this meant that Jonathan could continue to appeal even if I decided against it.

We had sent our penultimate letter to the Secretary of State for Health on 7 February 2002, asking him to reconsider if it was really proportionate to dispute our claim, given that they had already agreed to change the law. On 2 April, we gave notice of our application for judicial review and added myself as a litigant. Finally, on 17 April, we received a rather curt reply. They would indeed be opposing our action and, without giving us any specific reasons why, they abruptly denied that our human rights were being violated and/or that EC law had been breached.

I tried to put this to the back of my mind whilst I concentrated on the imminent arrival of my baby. I had been having a dilemma about whether to have a Caesarean section. There were no complications, but, having had my first child by Caesarean, I was advised that the chances of me getting through a natural birth without having to have an emergency operation in the middle of it were only around 60 per cent. If I had to be induced, the odds went down. I wanted to have a natural birth but didn't want to do anything that might endanger my child. I decided to have a Caesarean only if the baby would otherwise need inducing. A date was set for 10 July, almost a week after the baby's due date of 4 July. That way the theatre was already booked if the baby didn't arrive of its own accord.

For once, I felt quite organised and prepared. My bags were packed for the hospital. Liam had finally decided that he wanted a brother rather than a sister, and he spent his first night away from home as a practice for our arrangements for him to sleep over at his grandma and grandad Blood's whilst I was in hospital. I had even hired and trained someone to cover for my maternity leave at work, so I could relax and have the fullest opportunity to enjoy this special time.

Waiting for my labour to start was terribly exciting. As Liam had been delivered so early, I had missed this with my first pregnancy. Every night when I went to bed, I wondered if tonight would be the night. Every day was filled with an air of expectancy. Nothing happened.

Then suddenly, around eight o'clock one night, shortly after my due date, I felt a few twinges. I rang my parents and the hospital to tell them that I thought maybe it was time. I timed the contractions. They were around 20 minutes apart. I waited for them to get closer, but they didn't. After a couple of hours, they stopped altogether. It had been a false alarm.

I was booked in for an appointment the day before my planned Caesarean at the hospital, just to explain the procedure to me and to do any last-minute checks. I attended the appointment with a heavy heart, bitterly disappointed that my baby had not arrived naturally. I explained how I felt to the consultant and asked if it was possible to give it another week. He did a scan to check the baby still had enough fluid around it. Everything looked fine, so we decided to delay the Caesarean until 17 July.

Sadly, the extra week passed uneventfully, but at least I had peace of mind that I had given the baby the extra time. I am sure that God knows best. If my baby was to safely arrive naturally, with God's will I believe it could and would have done so.

I checked into hospital the evening before my operation. It was a different hospital to the one where Liam had been born because the old Jessop Hospital for Women had closed. The maternity provision was now a new extension, named the Jessop Wing after the old hospital, at the Royal Hallamshire, the very place where my husband had died and his sperm had been retrieved a little over seven years previously.

My parents and Liam came with me to get me settled in. It was a gloriously sunny day and we sat out on the hospital terrace while they carried out the various blood tests they needed and I filled in their questionnaires and consent forms. It seemed odd to me that there was so much to be done that had obviously been missed in the panic of Liam's birth. Finally, my parents left to take Liam to my in-laws' house.

My parents were going to come over first thing in the morning so Mum could come into the theatre with me. Gill and Brian were going to bring Liam over to see the baby as soon as it was born. I went to bed for the evening still hoping that maybe I'd go into labour that night, but I didn't.

The next morning, my Caesarean was delayed slightly, as the theatre was needed for an emergency. This didn't trouble me. I was just glad that I wasn't the emergency. Eventually, we were ready. I was taken into theatre and given a spinal anaesthetic, ready for the operation. Unfortunately, the anaesthetist had difficulty getting the needle into the right place on my back and it appeared not to have taken as well as it should have done. Everyone knew that I really didn't want to have a general anaesthetic, as I wanted to see my baby arrive. This was one of the reasons I had been so afraid of having an emergency operation. It was decided to give me an epidural as a sort of top-up. This meant that we were all in the theatre for ages whilst we waited first for one anaesthetic to take and then the second. My dad, who was outside, wondered what was happening. Eventually, we were ready and the consultant began the operation.

A green screen was placed across my tummy, but we had agreed beforehand that, when it was time to lift the baby out, the consultant would drop the screen altogether, so I could see the little one emerge.

I felt a bit of tugging and pushing and then the screen was removed. I strained to lift my head to witness a little bundle with a mass of dark hair being gently lifted from my tummy.

'It's a boy,' my mum told me.

I couldn't see because I was crying. He looked so beautiful. I held him briefly and then he was taken to be checked over by a paediatrician. He was perfect. This time my baby was fit and well, and could be handed straight back to me.

'Time of birth 10.57 a.m.,' the consultant recorded. 'What are you going to call him?'

I was still undecided between Joel Michael and Kyle Joseph. I had wanted to look at my baby's little face and decide which name seemed to fit the best. This was proving difficult because he was screaming so much that his tiny features were all screwed up. He was hungry and desperately rooted around for my nipples, which he soon found and sucked on with all his might. Unfortunately, my milk needed time to come in, so this didn't pacify him.

We were taken into a recovery room, where the nurse gave him his first bath and weighed him. He was 7 lb 13½ oz. Steph's parents then arrived with Liam, who was fascinated to see his baby brother. The nurse gave my baby some vitamin K on a spoon. It wasn't much like food, but it obviously did something to satisfy him, as he finally stopped screaming. At long last, we could all see how handsome he was. I decided to name him Joel Michael. I wondered if Steph would have approved of the choice. I knew that Liam liked the name, which was important to me. Steph was never far from my thoughts, but I concentrated more on my family who were there with me.

Apart from the abundance of black hair, Joel looked quite different to Liam as a baby. His face was much rounder than Liam's. He was a unique and perfect little human being.

My father released the news of his birth in time for the evening news, and the next day Andy Gallacher, the photographer who had photographed Liam shortly after his birth, came to photograph Joel. Once again, despite many offers from newspapers to do an exclusive deal, I decided to put the photographs on general release to everyone.

By the time we got home, much of the fuss had died down and I could enjoy my family in relative peace.

CHAPTER 24

Another day in court and another Private Member's Bill

Liam was so incredibly proud of his new baby brother and I am sure that Steph would have been too. Our first few weeks at home were lovely. Once again, my mum came to stay whilst I recovered from the Caesarean, but it was easier than the last time.

It was a warm summer, and Liam and I enjoyed taking Joel for walks to the local play park. Liam played on the slide whilst I sat on the seat watching him, Joel lying beside me in his pram. The other mothers would peer in and look.

'How old is he?' one asked.

'Six days,' I replied.

'Ah, come and look, he's brand new,' she called to her friend.

Brand new. Everything was brand new. I'll never forget my old life with Steph, but my boys were the future.

Many days we sat out on the patio, enjoying the sun with Gill, my mum and all those who came to visit and admire my new son.

Richard, the man covering for me at work, came round two mornings a week to discuss anything that needed addressing and I thought that all was going well. Then a bombshell landed. My two main clients, Mereway Kitchen and Bathrooms, and Clippasafe nursery products, both decided that they wanted to stop using my company on the basis that we had been formerly trading. I can't say I blame them. Since I had first begun working for them around ten years previously, they had both grown considerably.

Meanwhile, the time I could put into servicing their accounts was diminishing. All the same, it was totally unexpected and came as a shock. They had been part of my life for so long that I knew I would miss them dearly. Really, I should have gone out immediately and pitched for business in the same market areas, but, with Mereway, the news came less than six weeks since I'd had a baby. I still couldn't drive a car, let alone start a new business initiative. I decided to do less work and not to miss the irreplaceable time with my young family. Richard stayed on until the end of September and I still remain friends with my former clients.

I registered Joel's birth on the last available day that the law required me to do so. I knew that it was a task that had to be done, but I'd put it off because it wasn't something that I particularly relished the thought of. Not being allowed to name Joel's father turned what should have been an enjoyable experience into a mere administrative exercise. I felt cheated of the excitement that I ought to have felt.

Instead, I focused on the more cheerful task of, once again, printing postcards and writing to thank all those who had sent gifts, cards or letters of congratulations for Joel's birth whilst I was in the hospital. This time I also joined a post-natal group, which was something I had felt excluded from with Liam. With Joel, I felt more able to participate as a 'normal' mother. Even so, Victoria Beckham had just had another little boy named Romeo, and now that we both had two boys of almost exactly the same ages, I would still have liked to meet her.

Meanwhile, preparations were under way for Joel's baptism. I had given Liam such a grand party that I felt I had to place equal emphasis on Joel's. I didn't have quite as many guests, so I decided to do something slightly different to avoid too many comparisons. Instead of a marquee, we used a local hotel for the reception afterwards and I hired a jazz band to make it a lively, joyful occasion.

The big day, 27 October, finally arrived and the weather couldn't have been worse. Storms had been raging all night. The wind was howling and the rain lashed down in sheets. Reporters and photographers sat outside the church in their cars, waiting for us to arrive. I invited them into the church, as I could hardly leave them standing outside in such horrific weather.

The service passed with the usual ceremony. Joel was baptised with water from the colourful little font made by local schoolchildren. He was welcomed into the family of the church and I felt incredibly privileged to be the mother of such a handsome, sweet little boy. He still had masses of dark hair and a big, cheeky grin. He looked so beautiful in his little blue outfit and bootees embroidered with his name, the name of the church and date of his baptism.

We didn't allow photographs to be taken during the service. Instead, we had agreed to pose at the end. With all the reporters there, as well as family and friends, this took quite a while and our departure was delayed. Finally, though, we decided enough photographs had been taken. I spoke briefly to the reporters and then we piled into the cars and travelled in convoy to the Clumber Park Hotel for our buffet and celebration. When we arrived, the entrance to the car park was blocked. A huge oak tree lay across the path, so we had to go over the grass to reach the hotel.

I later learnt that the tree had fallen less than quarter of an hour before our arrival. If we hadn't been delayed, the chances are it would have landed on top of one of our cars. I wasn't too happy about the awful weather, but I think God must have been watching over us after all.

The day went with a swing. The jazz band were excellent and encouraged the children to join in, playing some little percussion instruments which they had brought with them. Liam thought it was great, particularly when they played his favourite song, 'Bear Necessities' from *Jungle Book*. Joel, meanwhile, enjoyed the attention of being passed around and shown off by his proud grandma and grandad Blood.

Many old friends came to join in the celebration, although sadly some of my guests had been prevented from travelling, whilst others were delayed. Fortunately, Michael Fordham, my barrister from my first court case, and his family had travelled up from the south the night before. He was now godfather to both my children. My solicitor, Richard Stein, and his family missed the church service but made it in time for the buffet. He sat on our table. We tried not to talk about my birth certificate case, but he assured me that the papers had been submitted to the court and we joked about Joel being one of the youngest litigants in history.

Another barrister, Tom De La Mare, was working on the case.

He had put in so much effort which was really beyond the call of duty that I felt that we too had become good friends. I had also invited him to Joel's baptism, but he had been unable to attend due to a prior engagement.

Following Joel's baptism celebrations, I suffered the same sense of loss that I had experienced immediately after Liam's. For about a week afterwards, I really missed being able to talk about the day with my husband. Steph was named as Liam and Joel's father on their baptism certificates, but not on their birth certificates.

A little under a month later, I was sitting at home when the fax machine rang and papers began to feed through. It was a letter from the Government's solicitors to mine. I began to read it. At first I couldn't believe my eyes and then I thought that perhaps I was interpreting it incorrectly. The Secretary of State for Health appeared to have given in. The letter acknowledged a breach of article 8 and/or article 8 read in conjunction with article 14 rights for all four litigants. We had argued that article 8, the right to private and family life, covered personal identity. Our submission was based on the fact that it included the right to choose or discover who one is (whether in genetic, social, ethnic, sexual or other terms) and then live in public accordingly. Article 14 provides that the rights and freedoms given by the Convention are non-discriminatory on any ground, including birth or other status.

I had barely read to the end of the letter before I called the solicitors.

'Does this mean what I think it does?'

I'm not sure that Richard Stein could quite believe it either.

'Yes, but it's not quite over yet,' he warned. 'The court still have to agree with you both and then you need the Minister to agree to amend the law by statutory instrument.'

I tried hard to be cautious and not to shout it from the rooftops. I was sure that the Government must be planning to amend the law by statutory instrument to have suddenly and dramatically made such a concession.

For this reason, I wasn't exactly over the moon when a reporter rang me at the beginning of December to tell me that Steve McCabe, MP for Birmingham Hall Green, had taken on my birth certificate Bill to bring forward as Private Member's legislation. It wasn't that I was ungrateful to him, just that I'd been there before and Private Member's Bills are so vulnerable to sabotage. As far as I was concerned, having the Bill amended by statutory instrument would have been a simpler option. Still, I didn't want my scepticism to reflect badly on Steve McCabe, so I tried to make the right noises to the reporter, whilst still remaining cautious.

Steve McCabe's new Human Fertilisation and Embryology (Deceased Fathers) Bill was printed on Liam's fourth birthday, 11 December 2002. It differed slightly from Tony Clarke's Bill, in that there were some new clauses about requiring written consent for future cases. This did not apply retrospectively, however, so Liam and Joel were still covered.

A court date was set for 28 February with Mr Justice Sullivan, the anniversary of the date I had initially asked for the sperm to be taken eight years before. We were listed for just 45 minutes, which sounded promising. If the judge was going to disagree that our situation was incompatible with the Human Rights Act, we thought he would have needed longer. The 45 minutes was needed to argue about costs and to try and set some parameters in relation to time so that we wouldn't be left waiting indefinitely for new legislation to be introduced once again. The new Private Member's Bill really meant that we couldn't push for an amendment by statutory instrument unless the Bill failed. However, if that should happen, we wanted the Government to have a finite amount of time in which to make their decision on whether to amend by this fast-track route, with leave to go back to the court if necessary. They would have rather left it all open-ended.

My whole family went to the Royal Courts of Justice. Sadly, Joanne Tarbuck could not attend because of particular work commitments on that day, which she couldn't evade.

Before the judge arrived, I took Liam into the courtroom to look around. He clung to my hand whilst taking in the unfamiliar details. The walls were lined with books and three huge chairs stood on a platform in front of him. The usher asked if he'd like to sit in the judge's chair, which he did.

Liam then joined Joel and my mum outside the courtroom whilst my dad and I went in to listen to the proceedings. It was quite a small room. I sat behind my solicitors to the rear and left of the room, near the door. The usual reporters filled the press seats which ran at a right angle to us, over to the right. In particular, I noted Joshua Rozenberg for the *Telegraph*. He was one of the two reporters who had first broken the news of my case when he'd worked for the BBC in 1996. He was still covering my story almost seven years later.

As he is a lawyer as well as a reporter, he was also one of probably only a couple of representatives from the media who managed to work out what on earth was going on. As it was still up to the judge to rule and I didn't want to tempt fate, I hadn't told anybody that the Government had given in, so they were all expecting an argument about the case itself. Instead, a declaration of incompatibility with the Human Rights Act 1998 on the terms we had agreed was granted almost immediately. The judge's only query was that he wanted to see the letter from Alan Milburn, the Secretary of State for Health, in which they had capitulated, as he appeared not to have it in his court bundle. He peered at it most quizzically through his narrow little reading glasses and then looked up.

'Extraordinary,' he declared.

Like myself, I don't think he could believe that my solicitors had written asking for precisely such an agreement immediately prior to us filing for action. Our opponents had refused and then, the minute we had pressed the go button, they had changed their mind, without any further evidence or arguments being presented in the interim.

We tried to find an explanation for this, but none was forthcoming. It was mainly on this basis that my solicitors had asked for our costs, which we estimated to be in the region of £20,000, to be repaid on an indemnity basis. Normally, when costs are awarded, as with my first court case, the applicant entitled to claim them would manage to recoup around 60 per cent of what they had paid, as they have to prove that it was legitimate and necessary. When costs are awarded on an indemnity basis, which is the highest level possible, the boot is on the other foot. If they dispute any costs, it is the defendant who must prove that it was not strictly necessary. The effect of this is that virtually all of the actual money spent can be recovered. It is extremely rare that costs are awarded on this basis and almost unheard of against a public body.

We were awarded costs at the normal level from the outset, but managed to get costs on an indemnity basis from the point that Tony Clarke's Private Member's Bill had collapsed. In the judge's view, this was when our threat to litigate became 'more serious'.

Justice Sullivan had already criticised the Department of Health, declaring it was 'not their most shining hour'. The unusual cost order further confirmed his displeasure at the way they had handled our claim. This was important because of the message it sent out, particularly as we were also granted leave to return to court if necessary. A time limit of two months was set for a decision on whether to amend the law by statutory instrument if Steve McCabe's Private Member's Bill failed.

I left the court feeling rather jubilant. At long last, I felt the end was in sight. Joanne rang me on my mobile the very second I turned it back on. I gave her the good news. I recorded some interviews with the amassed media just outside the Royal Courts of Justice and then went across the road to Blackstone Chambers, where our barrister, Tom De La Mare, worked. We wanted to take a few moments to debrief and celebrate, and also to meet up with Mike Fordham, my children's godfather, who had an office next to Tom's. Lord Lester's office was also just a few doors away, but he's a very busy man and sadly he wasn't in that day.

Mike couldn't have been more pleased if he'd argued the case himself. He recalled that, when he had first met me to discuss my first court case for the right to try for my late husband's child, he had warned me that, even if we won and I had a child, I would never get Stephen's name on the birth certificate. At the time, there was no domestic legal route to do so. I think his comment was that we had managed to achieve the 'virtually impossible', followed by the 'totally impossible'. This light-hearted praise was gratefully received by both myself and Tom. We posed whilst Mike took a couple of photos of us all, before heading home.

The second reading of Steve McCabe's Private Member's Bill passed relatively smoothly on 28 March 2003. It was an opportunity to meet the Bill's new champion for the first time and also to meet up once again with Tony Clarke, who was there to offer his support and to place on record in Hansard those private comments that Desmond Swayne had 'intervened under orders' when he had talked out his previous Bill. He wanted to make sure that nothing similar happened this time round.

The Committee stage was on Wednesday, 7 May. Once again, I travelled to London with my dad. We arrived a little late due to the incompatibility of train times and the early start for the proceedings. Sue Hayes, Steve McCabe's researcher, met us just inside the St Stephen's Gate entrance to Westminster and we were quickly ushered into the small Committee room. At the second reading, I had expressed some concerns to Steve McCabe that his Bill allowed no provision for anyone else to elect that the father be named on the birth certificate in the extremely unlikely event of the mother being unable to do so herself, for example if she died in childbirth or became temporarily incapacitated. He had tabled an amendment to deal with this. We arrived just in time to hear the amendment pass and then to hear Dr Evan Harris speak.

He had assured everyone at the third reading of Tony Clarke's Bill that his problems about lack of written consent were to do with future cases, but he now decided to question the Bill's retrospective provisions in that area too. Given that this could only relate to my family, I felt personally attacked. My father was seething and decided to take issue with Dr Harris when the Committee broke up. It all ended in a rather ugly exchange of words, whilst Hazel Blears, who had taken over Yvette Cooper's former position, looked on in absolute bemusement.

It is very frustrating to hear people talking about you and not to be able to answer back. They leave their mark on public records, but, if you get the chance at all, your response is limited to a few private remarks that are no doubt quickly forgotten by the individuals concerned. I offered to write to Dr Harris to explain why I believed his problems with the Bill could only apply to my family. The letter took me a good couple of days to write and was designed to help Dr Harris to understand things which he admitted he had little or no time to research. I asked if I had addressed his concerns but didn't receive the courtesy of a reply. I am sure that Dr Harris would claim that he was too busy. Apart from his work commitments, I later learnt that his partner was seriously ill. For that I am sorry, but I would like to have known if his concerns were satisfied before the third reading of the Bill on Friday, 13 June.

Now, I'm not a superstitious person, but we did joke about Friday the 13th perhaps not being the best day to have been given for such an important event. Initial indications were that it would be plain sailing, but we nearly ran aground due to the Fireworks Bill, which had its third reading before ours. There wasn't really any will to see it pass. It had become complicated due to the number of amendments and it looked likely to be talked out of time. If that happened, we wouldn't get onto our Bill and it would not pass. The whips worked very hard, trying to reach an agreement that would give our Bill the time it needed. In the end, they decided to let the Fireworks Bill go through as it was the only way to give ours a chance. They could always stop or further amend the Fireworks Bill in the Lords. Our Bill passed its final stage in the Commons. Dr Evan Harris wasn't in the House and we received good support from all those who spoke. We were all set for the Lords.

Baroness Pitkeathley gained the job of steering the Bill on its final voyage, but on 4 July, at its second reading in the Lords, many of my old supporters came out to help: Lord Winston, Baroness Warnock and, of course, Lord Lester all spoke eloquently on the Bill's behalf.

Joanne Tarbuck, Jan (her late husband's mother), myself and my father all had tickets below-bar to watch, which meant that we sat on the ground floor, right next to the chamber. Afterwards, we were invited by Lord Lester and Lord Winston for a drink in the Lords' bar. It was a shame that we hadn't brought the children because I would have loved to introduce them to Joel, but all the same it was good to be able to relax and reflect that soon it would all be over. We were assured that no one wished to amend the Bill at the Committee stage, meaning that the remainder of its passage was basically a formality.

The Bill had passed its second reading in the Lords on the day that Joel had been due to arrive the year previously, 4 July. There was supposed to be a minimum of a two-week gap before the next stage, taking it to 18 July, but Parliament rose for the summer recess on his first birthday, 17 July. The one extra day meant that we had to wait until the autumn, but I didn't really mind. At least now I could take my family on holiday knowing that I wouldn't miss the big day, and I was confident that the birth certificate Bill would pass and I wouldn't have to return to court.

CHAPTER 25

A name that made a difference

Liam broke up from nursery. We packed Joel's first birthday presents to take with us and, together with my parents, we headed off to Spain for a well-deserved break.

I played with my two boys, building sandcastles on the beach, listening to the waves lapping at the shore. Liam collected shells; Joel cheerfully raked patterns in the sand. A more tranquil and idyllic scene I could not have imagined. I thought back to the holidays that Steph and I had taken together and the turmoil of some of the intervening years. Finally, I felt that I had reclaimed my life.

Our apartment overlooked the sea. We were sitting out on the balcony later the same day when my mobile phone rang. It was a reporter from *Scotland on Sunday*. I was told that a paper had been printed in a 'well-respected' medical journal which claimed that retrieving my late husband's sperm was akin to rape and that it had been illegal and constituted an assault. It was written by academics who, although not from relevant fields, were from very credible institutions. One was a doctor from the School of Social Sciences at Glasgow Caledonian University, and the other a professor from the Frazer of Allander Institute, Department of Economics, University of Strathclyde. *Scotland on Sunday* was running an article on it that weekend.

I tried to respond as best as I could. The offending medical paper was faxed to a local hotel for me and I spent the evening poring over it. It made some outrageously incorrect claims. For a start, taking Steph's sperm was never found to be illegal and no one has been tried for assault, let alone been found guilty. *Scotland on Sunday* asked if I would be suing for defamation, but the medical journal, *Human Reproduction and Genetic Ethics*, told me their circulation was only between 200 and 250 for the whole of Europe. What would I achieve, even if I won? It's a pity the Scottish national newspaper gave the article further publicity, otherwise it might have ended there.

I asked the medical journal for the right to reply and spent two days writing my rebuttal, which they printed in full. They have since received a further response from the authors of the original article. The claims and counterclaims could go on for ever. At the time of writing this at the beginning of May 2004, I do not know whether the new reply will be printed. I have declined the opportunity to answer back. I can't keep looking over my shoulder and jumping to the defence of my family. I am not an academic. The prestige of achieving publication in such a journal doesn't gain me the admiration of my peers or help either directly or indirectly to pay my bills.

The whole sorry episode made me realise that it will never be over and my life can never be my own unless I am prepared to ignore all that is written or said about my family. History is being rewritten by the academics and the 'experts', yet not one of them lived it, breathed it and had nightmares over it as I did. Even those who were more closely involved, like Ruth Deech, did not appear to know the details as well as me. After my case had finished, she commented that the 'quality of the sperm remained to be seen', meaning she was unsure if it was viable enough to achieve a pregnancy. At the time, I found this a bit strange, as I had submitted evidence as to the quality of the sperm at the very outset. I knew the evidence presented by the HFEA back to front and I expected her to know mine in the same detail. However, in hindsight, I don't suppose she had the same emotional investment in the outcome that I did. To her, it was just one case. To me, it was my life.

I have even met former members of the HFEA who served on the committee at the time of my case. They have tried to assure me that some of them really did try to look at my case compassionately, but 'the law was the law'. They obviously have still missed the point. It wasn't the law, otherwise I would not have won my appeal. They refused to meet with either myself or my lawyers, so they never heard my side of the legal argument.

The national press coverage from my case doesn't worry me, because, by and large, the papers adhere to a code which means they must contact the person concerned to give them a chance to reply and that they must give fairly even coverage of all sides of an argument. Those who later profess to be experts, with no real basis for their claim except for perhaps a few letters after their name, trouble me no end.

I recently helped some law undergraduates who were doing a project about my case. They had researched it well and I was amazed to see the bibliography included so many articles and books written since my case which obviously refer to us in reasonable detail. Their references even included a book by Ruth Deech. I haven't the faintest idea whether all of these are accurate or not. What I can be sure of is that the details they have chosen to highlight will be those which best reflect the author's view and, if I read them, I would probably wish to add some points of my own. Sure, I can choose not to look at them, but Liam and Joel may one day do so. I fear what they may find, particularly as the mists of time begin to blur the truth. I want them to know what really happened, not some diluted interpretation presented as an independent report, yet designed to convey a particular opinion.

I welcomed the chance to speak at a conference organised by the British Infertility Counselling Association. It gave me the opportunity to counsel the profession that had spent so much time counselling me, and I think it is a wise and brave move to seek the opinion of former patients. I have also taken part in a cross-continental video debate with medical and ethical professionals organised by Imperial College, London. This was very interesting and gave me the chance to catch up with Lord Winston, who was chairing the proceedings, and also to meet Professor Sheila McLean, who had written the review of the law commissioned because of my case. After all, it was Professor McLean who had recommended that the law in relation to birth certificates be changed, even if she didn't mention anything about making it retrospective. To an extent, I feel that I have intruded into the small world of these distinguished professionals, but I am a temporary guest.

A name that made a difference

I also try to help some potential patients who call me and ask for my advice. Sometimes I have declined to get involved because of the impact it would have on my own family. One lady asked if I would donate eggs because she had no one to help her and it was the only way she could get further up the waiting list at her chosen fertility clinic. I doubt I'd have considered it anyway, but I was breastfeeding, so it was impossible. I told her about egg-sharing, where she could pay for another woman's treatment cycle in return for half of her eggs. Her clinic didn't sanction those kind of schemes, however, and she seemed very afraid of suggesting or doing anything that may upset them. Fertility specialists and nurses hold huge sway over the lives of those who place their hopes and dreams in their hands, and patients appear to be afraid of changing clinics for fear they might lose what little they already have. In this case, the woman was afraid of losing her place on the waiting list at one clinic by looking into the possibilities afforded by trying somewhere else. When you are already feeling vulnerable, the pressure to conform with a particular clinic's view can be overwhelming, even if it is not intentional.

It therefore upset me greatly when a British woman lost her High Court appeal to gain access to treatment with her late husband's sperm, when she claimed that the clinic had placed her husband under duress to make him alter his permission for her to use his sperm after his death, should the totally unexpected happen. The clinic admitted it was their policy to encourage people to change their minds in such a case and the man would be asked to withdraw his consent.

With other couples the consent has not been withdrawn, but may be in the form of a letter. At the time of my court case, many people wrote to me saying that they had taken it upon themselves to express their wishes in this form. Some clinicians appear unsure whether this is a satisfactory method of recording consent, but the law only requires the consent to be in writing. It does not specify that it needs to be on a certain form. There is a requirement for the opportunity to receive counselling, but it is not mandatory to receive any. If the man had wanted to receive counselling, he could have done so at the time he wrote the letter. To me, it seems far more relevant that his widow be counselled after his death.

I was pleased to see in November 2003 that Israel issued a new directive which allows posthumous conception by wives and life-partners, unless the deceased had made expressions to the contrary during their lifetime. I would like this to be the case in Britain, but, even though the whole fertility law is currently under review, I hold no hope that this will happen, as the review by Professor Sheila McLean did not recommend it. I would, however, still like to see increased flexibility in the law in general, allowing more decisions to be made on a case-by-case basis.

Fertility law is also under review across the other side of the world in Victoria, Australia, where they are specifically addressing the question of posthumous conception. Their mind has been focused on this due to the case there relating to a widow known as 'AB'. The Australian woman involved has recently visited me on two occasions to gain help and insight into the legal arguments used in my case. Her husband died in 1998 and she obtained a Supreme Court order for permission to retrieve his sperm but has been refused permission to use or export it to another state. Her problem is that her husband died in Victoria, one of only two states in Australia which, on the face of it, appear to prohibit the procedure. She is kind and good with my children. She works for a relief agency, caring for others, but tells few of her own problems. She has degrees in fine art, social work and a masters in international development. She is an intelligent lady. She still pursues this path after such a long time because she knows it is right and what her husband would have wanted. I have tried to assist, but I am frustrated that I can do so little to relieve a suffering I know so well.

I don't have all the answers. I do the best I know how. We have no secrets in our home. Liam and Joel visit their father's grave and Liam knows that they both share the same daddy, who sadly died before they were in their mummy's tummy. He doesn't understand any specific importance in the fact that their father died before they were conceived, as opposed to merely dying before they were born. He is sad that he didn't have the opportunity to know his daddy, but not unduly so, and he has a secret little smile when his grandma Blood passes comment that some of his mannerisms are 'just like his dad'. He is also fascinated by old photographs of Steph, although no more so than photos of myself when I was younger. These are not hidden away and we still have a couple of wedding photos on display in frames around our home.

My children's situation is not the same as those who do not know who their father is and we are not a single-parent family in the same sense as those which have been disrupted by divorce or separation. Liam and Joel are assured that their parents loved one another deeply and we all have the full support of loving paternal relations. Steph may be absent, but he is still a part of our children's lives, both through his family and because their father's views and wishes filter through into their upbringing. Occasionally, when I find myself shouting at them, I hear Steph's voice, reminding me to be more tolerant. Once, when Liam was very young, he decided to pull the petals off the flowers we were putting on Steph's grave. My initial anger was checked, as Steph wouldn't have minded, any more than he'd have minded them putting stickers all over their bedroom units. I remember teasing him about that when he was lovingly fitting the units just a few days before he fell ill. I said that they wouldn't look so good if our child decided to decorate them with stickers; Steph disagreed. He thought that kids should be allowed to be kids.

Liam now has several posters and school certificates Blu-tacked to those same units. He is a thoughtful and extremely sensitive child. I remember Dame Jill Knight in the House of Commons saying that a sensitive child would have nightmares about the circumstances of their birth, if they were conceived in the manner I proposed. Once Liam did have a bad dream, but it wasn't about his father, just the usual stuff which troubles children as they lie alone at night in a darkened room. I am far more likely to hear Liam chuckling away to himself in his sleep, with an angelic smile spread across his face.

If anyone asks Liam about his father, he responds confidently. So far, Liam's only problem appears to be that he has had to accept that death is a part of life at an earlier age than most of his peers. We live in a society which shields children from death. Mostly they are absent from funerals and are told that people die (especially mummies and daddies) only when they are very old. Our family cannot live with the luxury of this lie, but Liam doesn't worry excessively, as he readily accepts my alternative explanation that we'll all remain on this earth as long as God has a purpose for us to be here and it is part of His plan.

Learning about death at an early age does have some advantages. Liam appreciates that our time here is very precious.

Until you realise that it will one day come to an end, it is hard to fully appreciate the gift of life or to be party to the mourning of those who go before us.

Recently we lost an elderly neighbour. Liam accompanied me to the memorial church service. He wanted to go. At the beginning of the service, I wondered if I had done the right thing to take him. Initially, he wept buckets and, like any mother, I didn't like to see my son upset. However, with hindsight, I am confident that it was the right thing to do. I think that if I had not taken him, it might have protected me from seeing my little boy cry but not done anything to cushion Liam. The service was a real celebration of life, by a vicar we know, at the church we attend every week. Liam understands that he was not alone in feeling sad that our neighbour had died and now readily accepts that he has gone to heaven. It is an open subject that we can talk about, not something to be shelved for discussion later.

It is a shame for us (although understandable for them) that this is not the case in most families with such young children. Shortly after Liam first started school, I was suddenly faced with a barrage of questions relating to life, death and possibly the circumstances of his birth: 'How did God make me? What am I made out of? Why do people die? Can Daddy see me? Where exactly in the sky is heaven?'

At first I was suspicious as to what had triggered this sudden inquisitiveness, but then I realised that Liam was just trying to answer the questions that other children asked of him. If they asked about his dad, he explained that he didn't have one because he'd died. Liam then became the 'expert' on the subject. But, of course, he wasn't, so he came home every night and asked me. I tried to be truthful and told him that I didn't know all the answers either. I offered my view, whilst telling him that others may think differently. After about a week, the questions stopped. The playground chatter had obviously moved on to a different subject.

Occasionally, it crops up again. One night when I picked Liam up from school, he rushed out and asked, 'Mummy, how old was Daddy when he died?'

'Thirty,' I replied, 'but, darling, why do you ask?'

He didn't hear my question, as he'd run off to tell his friend.

She frowned, 'You don't die when you're 30.' Her response was directed more at me than Liam.

A name that made a difference

I didn't know what to say. I didn't want to contradict anything her parents might have told her, so we made a rapid escape. Liam was very upset by this episode. Not realising that Liam's father was no longer with us, two of Liam's closest little friends had asked some innocent question about his father shortly before home time. Liam explained that he had died, but it was a long time ago, before he was in his mummy's tummy. The children didn't believe that his father was dead. It is one of the 'golden rules' at Liam's school that you should always tell the truth. What reduced Liam to tears was not the death of his father but the fact that his friends thought he was lying.

This, combined with the inaccurate accounts that have been printed about my family, made me realise that I needed to set the record straight once and for all, if not for myself then for my children. The truth is like a well-cut diamond. It should be clear, but it has many facets and reflects differently depending on which side you look at. This is unashamedly my story. It is the truth as I saw it, as I lived it, at the time.

As for the future, those pages have yet to be written. It would be possible to have more children by Steph, but, given the difficulty I had conceiving Joel, I doubt I'd be successful even if I tried. I might like to find another soulmate to share my life with, but I suspect that I've been through rather too much alone. Steph was a strong person, a real emotional support to me. After everything I've been through, this is a tough position to fill. The right person may be able to enhance our lives, but my experiences have taught me to appreciate what I have. I am very happy with my family and, because I still feel the glow from the love that Steph and I once shared, I do not particularly feel that anything is missing.

Our birth certificate Bill finally completed its passage through Parliament on 18 September 2003. Liam took the day off school to join myself, Joel and my parents, as we attended the House of Lords for its final reading. Joanne and Jonathan Tarbuck went along with their family, and also Marian Jordan with her posthumously conceived son, Daniel. Although Marian was not party to our litigation, she too had been active in campaigning for the law to be changed and, unlike Joanne and myself, had in fact refused to register her son's birth altogether until she could name his father on the certificate.

Jonathan was old enough to sit in the public gallery at the House of Lords, but we had been told that the other children were too young to be allowed in. We had planned for them to remain in Peers' lobby, just outside the chamber. Joanne, myself and our respective fathers again had seats 'below-bar'. Marian, who had also brought along her brother in case she needed someone to look after Daniel, finally managed to get all of her family into a special gallery allotted to MPs. Liam and Joel were the only ones left outside with my mother.

There was some discussion about hereditary peers scheduled for that day, so the House of Lords was packed. Liam and Joel enjoyed meeting the many important people as they made their way into the chamber. Many stopped to admire them and tell my mother how they remembered me being there before they were born. One of the doormen on duty that day was called Mr Blood. I remembered meeting him before. I could hardly forget, when we both shared the same name.

We knew that our Bill was to be read very early in the proceedings and that it would all be over in a matter of seconds. There was so much business to get through on that day that there was no time for anyone to say anything beyond the formalities. The House looked splendid. It was full to overflowing. We sat only inches from Margaret Thatcher, and the gold and red decor glistened under the lights. I was sorry that Liam was to miss such a spectacle, so when one of the doormen came in to tell me that a reporter had requested to see me outside, I grabbed my opportunity to ask him if he could possibly bring Liam in to join me for the few seconds whilst the Human Fertilisation and Embryology (Deceased Fathers) Bill was read. He said he'd see what he could do.

Shortly afterwards, he appeared with Liam. I went and sat at the back with my four-year-old son and whispered that he had to keep very quiet and remember what he saw. Liam never made a murmur. His mouth fell slightly open and his eyes grew wide as they moved slowly around the chamber. I think that he took away a sense of importance, although clearly he did not understand the relevance of the few words uttered by Baroness Pitkeathley that signalled that our birth certificate Bill had finally made it through Parliament. Unusually, a session of Royal Assent was scheduled for later that same day, so we knew that by the evening our law would be on the statute books. There would then be a period of around two months before it came into force.

A name that made a difference

Afterwards, my family celebrated in the Lords' bar with Baroness Pitkeathley, Steve McCabe, Sue Hayes (his researcher) and Joanne Tarbuck's family. Unfortunately, we didn't have long because I had appointments with reporters outside. Many of them had followed my story from the very beginning and I owed it to them to see it through to the final chapter. We posed briefly on the steps of Westminster and then went across the road to the green just opposite. I'd been there many times before, standing before the microphones and cameras. This day was different. The sun shone brilliantly and we were relaxed and happy. I sat down on the grass with my children to pose, as requested. Liam leant against me, almost pushing Joel and myself over. We collapsed in heaps of laughter.

Once the photo call and interviews were over, we met up again with Joanne Tarbuck and her family in the park just next to Westminster. We took some photos of our own, and the children played happily, throwing the fallen autumnal leaves that covered the floor. Liam and Jonathan chased each other and Joel trotted along giggling some distance behind them. He didn't realise that he'd never catch them. Joel thought that he was joining in the big boys' game, although I doubt that Liam or Jonathan noticed until they finally stopped to catch their breath.

We went home the following day and Gill, my mother-in-law, gave me a big hug as soon as she saw me.

'That's for finally getting it through,' she said.

She didn't need to say any more. I knew that once Liam had been born, getting Stephen's name (she never called him Steph) on his children's birth certificates had been of utmost importance to her.

On 1 December 2003, the Human Fertilisation and Embryology Act 2003 came into force. I went along to Sheffield registry office to re-register Liam and Joel's births that very morning. Sheffield City Council kindly gave me copies of their new birth certificates free of charge.

Liam Stephen Blood and Joel Michael Blood now officially have two parents.

Mother: Diane Michelle Blood. Occupation: Copywriter

Father: Stephen Brian Blood. Occupation: Kitchen and Bathroom Installations Manager (deceased).

Even though Steph died at 30, he has at least realised some of his wishes relayed to me shortly before his death. He got the funeral he wanted, packed with mourners, and he will be remembered not only by his children (who are told about him) but because he has made his mark on history. His existence changed the constitution of Britain and arguably left the world a better place. Maybe not for many, but for a few children he made a difference. From now on, children conceived after their father's death can have their deceased parent registered from the outset. If Steph could have changed things for anyone, it is children he would have chosen. If he could have chosen the means, love would be the answer. Without his inspiration and the warmth of that love, I could never have achieved our goals.

Steph even got me to write that book he'd always encouraged me to do. I expect it may cause criticism from some quarters, on the grounds that it may harm the welfare of my children. I have considered this but have concluded that, given what has already happened, their interests are best served by choosing to publish it.

You now know me and my late husband a little better, but you do not know my children. Whilst I have discussed a few relevant issues in relation to their father, I have taken great care to tread as lightly as possible on their privacy. This is the flesh on the bones of a story that is already a matter of public record. It is both my personal account for Liam and Joel, and my assurance that the wider world knows what they will learn about their origins. At five years old, Liam already knows what it has taken me thirty-eight years to realise: it is most hurtful when your testimony is contradicted by those with less access to the facts than yourself.

Gone is the searing pain which once ripped me apart, leaving me feeling as though the raw flesh were exposed from my stomach, but not always the sense that my family is discussed without regard to my human emotion. Just as I once pleaded with the HFEA to remember that 'I am a real human being', I now ask others to consider that too. At the end of it all, I am flesh and blood. My husband and I were 'one flesh'. We have two wondrous children, Liam and Joel Blood. They are our flesh. They are our blood, both in name and through the genetic ties that bind us.